TRANSCULTURAL COMMUNICATION IN HEALTH CARE

Joan Luckmann, RN, MA

Contributing Author

Sylvia Tindell Nobles, CRNP, MSN

Director, Medical Assisting
Trenholm State Technical College
Adjunct Faculty, School of Nursing
Auburn University at Montgomery
Montgomery, Alabama

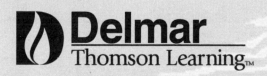

Delmar
Thomson Learning™

Africa • Australia • Canada • Denmark • Japan • Mexico
New Zealand • Phillipines • Puerto Rico • Singapore • Spain
United Kingdom • United States

NOTICE TO THE READER

Publisher does not warrant or guarantee any of the products described herein or perform any independent analysis in connection with any of the product information contained herein. Publisher does not assume, and expressly disclaims, any obligation to obtain and include information other than that provided to it by the manufacturer.

The reader is expressly warned to consider and adopt all safety precautions that might be indicated by the activities described herein and to avoid all potential hazards. By following the instructions contained herein, the reader willingly assumes all risks in connection with such instructions.

The publisher makes no representations or warranties of any kind, including but not limited to, the warranties of fitness for particular purpose or merchantability, nor are any such representations implied with respect to the material set forth herein, and the publisher takes no responsibility with respect to such material. The publisher shall not be liable for any special, consequential, or exemplary damages resulting, in whole or in part, from the readers' use of, or reliance upon, this material.

Delmar Staff:

Business Unit Director: William Brottmiller
Executive Editor: Cathy L. Esperti
Developmental Editor: Darcy M. Scelsi
Executive Marketing Manager: Dawn F. Gerrain
Project Editor: Elizabeth B. Keller
Production Coordinator: James Zayicek

Printed in Canada
4 5 6 7 8 9 10 XXX 05 04

For more information, contact Delmar, 3 Columbia Circle, PO Box 15015, Albany, NY 12212-0515; or find us on the World Wide Web at http://www.delmar.com

Library of Congress Cataloging-in-Publication Data

Luckmann, Joan.
    Transcultural communication in health care / Joan Luckmann; contributing author,
Sylvia Tindell Nobles.
        p. cm.
    Includes bibliographical references and index.
    ISBN 0-7668-0593-X -- ISBN 0-7668-0593-X
    1. Transcultural medical care. I. Nobles, Sylvia Tindell. II. Title.
    [DNLM: 1. Health Personnel. 2. Communication. 3. Cross-Cultural Comparison. 4.
Professional-Patient Relations. W 21 L941t 2000]
    RA418.5.T73 L83 2000
    362.1--dc21

                                                                            99-040689

Dedication

For my father
Ramon Romero
(1905-1980)

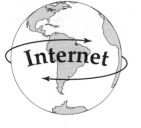

CONTENTS

PREFACE

Transcultural Communication in Health Care is designed to help you—the health care student—excel in today's multicultural health care workplace by improving your transcultural communication skills. This practical textbook will enable you to recognize and overcome cultural biases, learn about different styles of communication, and develop the transcultural communication skills you must have to communicate clearly with clients and health care providers from diverse cultures.

Successful transcultural communication is a skill that requires specific knowledge, training, and practice. To communicate confidently with clients and health care professionals from other cultures, it is important to (1) learn about the beliefs and values of different cultural groups, (2) recognize the barriers to transcultural communication, and (3) practice a variety of transcultural communication techniques. Because the population of the United States is becoming more culturally diverse, there is an urgent need to develop your transcultural communication skills. Use *Transcultural Communication in Health Care* to guide you as you study, and then practice transcultural communication techniques in the health care workplace.

ORGANIZATION AND CONTENT

Transcultural Communication in Health Care is organized into five units. Each unit opens with a self-assessment section and closes with a self-evaluation section. The self-assessment and self-evaluation exercises are structured to help you identify cultural biases and prejudices, overcome communication barriers, and develop your own communication style.

Unit One: Exploring Transcultural Communication focuses on concepts that are the prerequisites for developing transcultural communication skills. This unit builds on the fundamental principle that all individuals have cultural traditions that influence their patterns of interaction and communication. The chapters in Unit One will help you recognize that your interactions with clients represent the values of your culture, the values of the health care

xi

subculture, and your clients' culturally-influenced values and communication styles.

Specifically, the chapters in this unit discuss:

- The growing demand for transcultural communication in health care settings.

- Building blocks that form the basis for transcultural communication: culture, cultural values, beliefs, behavior, and communication.

- Stumbling blocks that impede transcultural communication: lack of knowledge, fear and distrust, racism, bias, ethnocentrism, stereotyping, ritualistic behavior, language barriers, and conflicting perceptions and expectations.

- Interactions between health care system subcultures that may positively or negatively affect transcultural communication; for example interactions between Western health care, hospital, health care professional and client subcultures.

Unit Two: Developing Transcultural Communication Skills concentrates on helping you to develop your observational, listening, nonverbal, and verbal transcultural communication skills. Unit Two offers practical suggestions for developing relationships with clients from different cultures by conveying empathy, showing respect, building trust, establishing rapport, listening actively, and providing appropriate feedback. This unit gives specific directions in how to:

- Explore transcultural situations as a participant–observer by interacting with people from different cultures as they go about their normal lives; for example, exploring ethnic neighborhoods and attending family celebrations and religious ceremonies.

- Establish a therapeutic relationship and communication with clients from diverse cultures.

- Overcome transcultural communication barriers.

- Communicate with clients who are not proficient in English, with or without the help of a professional interpreter.

- Work successfully with professional medical interpreters.

Unit Three: Using Transcultural Communication to Elicit Assessment Data and Develop Interventions builds on the important premise that a thorough cultural assessment of the client forms the basis for culturally-appropriate interventions. One goal of transcultural communication is to decrease the imposition of Western health care values on clients when these values hinder clients from achieving their own health objectives. By carefully assessing clients and learning more about their perspective, you should be able to (1) decrease transcultural conflicts, (2) evaluate the client's culturally influenced needs, (3) determine the client's health needs, and (4) arrive at a mutually agreeable plan of care.

Specifically, Unit Three should help you to:

- Develop the art of eliciting culturally-related information from clients.

- Ask questions that will elicit the client's perspective on illness, as well as the viewpoints of the client's family and support group.

- Formulate and write culturally-appropriate interventions that are based on a culturally-competent assessment.

- Inspire other health care professionals to use and promote culturally-appropriate interventions.

Unit Four: Using Transcultural Communication To Plan And Implement Care moves from how to perform a cultural assessment to how to use transcultural communication for planning care, teaching clients, and providing care. This unit provides:

- Techniques for developing plans of care that are tailored to meet the client's cultural perceptions and expectations.

- Techniques for assessing the learning needs of clients from other cultures.

- Techniques for teaching clients from other cultures about prescribed medications, procedures, hospital policies, life style changes that they may need to make, and home care.

- Techniques for assisting clients and families from other cultures cope with pain, grief, dying, and death.

You may wonder: "How can I possibly learn enough about all the different cultural groups to plan for, care for, and instruct my clients?" Remember that it is not necessary to know in detail the values and expected behaviors of different cultural groups. It **is** important to learn about each client's cultural perception of illness and health care, as well as each client's culturally determined expectations for care.

Unit Five: Transcultural Communication Skills Between Health Care Professionals focuses on communication between health care professionals in the health care workplace, which is often a multinational, multicultural setting.

This unit presents:

- Major barriers that impede transcultural communication between health care professionals from different cultures; for example, clashes in values and language differences.

- Different approaches you can use to improve your transcultural communication with physicians, and other health care professionals from different cultures.

- Techniques for the health care manager who identifies conflicts among workers and tensions between health care professionals and clients.

SPECIAL FEATURES

Special features of this book include the following exercises, techniques, tests, boxes, and resources:

- **Self-assessment exercises** are at the beginning of each unit. These exercises are designed to increase self-awareness; identify underlying attitudes, biases, and prejudices that can block your transcultural communication; and assess your transcultural communication style.

- **Self-evaluation exercises** are at the end of every unit. These exercises will help to evaluate your progress as you proceed through the chapters in each unit.

- **Transcultural Communication Diary**, included in the self-assessment and self-evaluation exercises, will allow you to record, analyze, and cultivate the transcultural communication insights and skills you are learning about in each unit.

- **Key Terms** at the beginning of every chapter list the 8–10 concepts that are central to comprehending the chapter. You should understand the terms and their relevance to transcultural communication after completing each chapter.

- **Learning Objectives** at the beginning of each chapter will encourage you to focus on the key concepts, strategies, and approaches that are addressed in the chapter content.

- **Step-by-step transcultural communication techniques**, using real world scenarios, are located throughout the book. These techniques provide clear directions for improving your communication with clients and health care professionals from other cultures.

- **Communication Considerations** boxes serve to highlight important information about transcultural communication.

- **Testing Your Knowledge** multiple-choice tests are found at the end of every chapter. A Test Answer Key is located in Appendix III.

- **Organizations and Agencies** that provide transcultural information and resources are located in Appendix I. These resources include professional organizations, government agencies, ethnic and minority organizations, international agencies, refugee centers, and telephone information lines.

- **Annotated lists of suggested books and films** with a transcultural theme are located in Appendix II. These books (fiction and non-fiction) and films demonstrate communication between cultures, and they have been selected to enhance your understanding of transcultural interaction.

ACKNOWLEDGMENTS

I wish to thank the following talented and dedicated people who participated in the writing, development, and production of this book:

Margaret A. McKenna, PhD, RN for developing the original continuing education course *Transcultural Communication in Nursing,* and for contributing her impressive knowledge of transcultural nursing to the introductory chapter for this book.

I also wish to thank the following people at Delmar:

William Brottmiller, Publisher, for recognizing the need for this book, and giving me the opportunity to develop the project.

Cathy Esperti, Executive Editor, for her keen insights and helpful suggestions, and ever present encouragement.

Darcy Scelsi, Developmental Editor, for her support and good humor, and for helping me with the many details that are a part of writing a book.

Tim Conners, Art and Design Coordinator, for designing an elegant format and book.

I would also like to thank the others who helped with the book:

Judi Orozco for always being available to discuss questions and concerns, and for expediting production.

Cynthia Roat, Interpreter Training Coordinator, for her careful review of Chapter 9: Working With and Without an Interpreter, and her excellent suggestions.

Dawn Gerrain, Executive Marketing Manager, for championing the marketing vision and materials for the book.

Lydia DeSantis, PhD, RN, FAAN, for contributing Chapter 6: Exploring Transcultural Communication As A Participant Observer, and for her help in suggesting books and films with a transcultural theme for Appendix II.

Oneida Hughes, PhD, RN, for contributing Chapter 12: Using Transcultural Communication to Assist People Responding To Pain, Grief, Dying, and Death.

Carol Leppa, PhD, RN, for contributing Chapter 5: Transcultural Communication Within The Health Care Subculture.

Royale Landy for her friendship, support, and help throughout the preparation of the original continuing education course and this book.

Chris Luckmann for his creative ideas and encouragement throughout the process of developing the manuscript.

Kelly Doran, MLS, for her excellent library research.

The reviewers who contributed their time and their suggestions for improving the manuscript.

Finally, I want to thank all of the patients, health care professionals, and health educators from diverse cultures who, over the years, have helped me to recognize the true and growing need for this timely and relevant book—*Transcultural Communication in Health Care*.

CONTRIBUTORS

Margaret A. McKenna, PhD, MPH, MN
University of Washington
Seattle, Washington

Carol J. Leppa, RN, PhD
University of Washington
Seattle, Washington

Lydia DeSantis, PhD, RN, FAAN
University of Miami
Coral Gables, Florida

Oneida M. Hughes, PhD, RN
Texas Woman's University
Dallas, Texas

UNIT ONE

EXPLORING TRANSCULTURAL COMMUNICATION

1

UNIT ONE
ASSESSMENT

ASSESSING YOUR TRANSCULTURAL COMMUNICATION GOALS AND BASIC KNOWLEDGE

Exercise One: Assessing Your Personal Objectives

What is your objective for studying transcultural communication? Check those points listed below that apply to you or write down your own objectives.

My personal objectives are to:

_____ Learn about the effects of culture on communication.

_____ Identify my own patterns of communication that have been influenced by my culture.

_____ Develop skill in identifying clients' different cultural beliefs.

_____ Decrease the frustration I experience when working with clients whose primary language is not English.

_____ Improve my effectiveness in conveying information to clients from different cultures.

_____ Overcome cultural biases that are blocking my ability to relate well to clients from different cultural backgrounds.

_____ Sharpen my skills in assessing clients who speak little English and who have different cultural values from my own.

_____ Improve my ability to convey health information to clients from different cultures.

_____ Give more culturally sensitive care.

My other objectives for studying this book are to: _____

_____

_____

Exercise Two: Assessing How You Relate To Various Groups of People in Society

The following self-test questionnaire will help you to assess how you relate to various groups of people in society. This in turn will help you to assess how you relate to various groups of clients in your care. Take a moment now to complete and score this test.

SELF-TEST QUESTIONNAIRE

How Do You Relate to Various Groups of People in Society?

Described below are different levels of response you might have toward a person.

Levels of Response:
1. *Greet:* I feel I can greet this person warmly and welcome him or her sincerely.
2. *Accept:* I feel I can honestly accept this person as he or she is and be comfortable enough to listen to his or her problems.
3. *Help:* I feel I would genuinely try to help this person with his or her problems as they might relate to or arise from the label/stereotype given to him or her.
4. *Background:* I feel I have the background of knowledge and/or experience to be able to help this person.
5. *Advocate:* I feel I could honestly be an advocate for this person.

The following is a list of individuals. Read down the list and place a check mark by anyone you would not "greet or would hesitate to greet." Then move to response level 2, "accept," and follow the same procedure. Try to respond honestly, not as you think might be socially or professionally desirable. Your answers are only for your personal use in clarifying your initial reactions to different people.

Level of Response Individual	1 Greet	2 Accept	3 Help	4 Background	5 Advocate
1. Haitian	☐	☐	☐	☐	☐
2. Child abuser	☐	☐	☐	☐	☐
3. Jew	☐	☐	☐	☐	☐
4. Person with hemophilia	☐	☐	☐	☐	☐
5. Neo-Nazi	☐	☐	☐	☐	☐
6. Mexican American	☐	☐	☐	☐	☐
7. IV drug user	☐	☐	☐	☐	☐
8. Catholic	☐	☐	☐	☐	☐
9. Senile, elderly person	☐	☐	☐	☐	☐
10. Teamster Union member	☐	☐	☐	☐	☐
11. Native American	☐	☐	☐	☐	☐

(continues)

Level of Response Individual	1 Greet	2 Accept	3 Help	4 Background	5 Advocate
12. Prostitute	☐	☐	☐	☐	☐
13. Jehovah's Witness	☐	☐	☐	☐	☐
14. Cerebral palsied person	☐	☐	☐	☐	☐
15. E.R.A. proponent	☐	☐	☐	☐	☐
16. Vietnamese American	☐	☐	☐	☐	☐
17. Gay/Lesbian	☐	☐	☐	☐	☐
18. Atheist	☐	☐	☐	☐	☐
19. Person with AIDS	☐	☐	☐	☐	☐
20. Communist	☐	☐	☐	☐	☐
21. Black American	☐	☐	☐	☐	☐
22. Unmarried expectant teen	☐	☐	☐	☐	☐
23. Protestant	☐	☐	☐	☐	☐
24. Amputee	☐	☐	☐	☐	☐
25. Ku Klux Klansman	☐	☐	☐	☐	☐
26. White Anglo-Saxon	☐	☐	☐	☐	☐
27. Alcoholic	☐	☐	☐	☐	☐
28. Amish person	☐	☐	☐	☐	☐
29. Person with cancer	☐	☐	☐	☐	☐
30. Nuclear armament proponent	☐	☐	☐	☐	☐

Scoring Guide: The previous activity may help you anticipate difficulty in working with some clients at various levels. The 30 types of individuals can be grouped into five categories: ethnic/racial, social issues/problems, religious, physically/mentally handicapped, and political. Transfer your checkmarks to the following form. If you have a concentration of checks within a specific category of individuals or at specific levels, this may indicate a conflict that could hinder you from rendering effective professional help.

Level of Response Individual	1 Greet	2 Accept	3 Help	4 Background	5 Advocate
Ethnic/Racial					
1. Haitian American	☐	☐	☐	☐	☐
6. Mexican American	☐	☐	☐	☐	☐
11. Native American	☐	☐	☐	☐	☐
16. Vietnamese American	☐	☐	☐	☐	☐
21. Black American	☐	☐	☐	☐	☐
26. White Anglo Saxon	☐	☐	☐	☐	☐
Social Issues/Problems					
2. Child abuser	☐	☐	☐	☐	☐
7. IV drug user	☐	☐	☐	☐	☐
12. Prostitute	☐	☐	☐	☐	☐
17. Gay/Lesbian	☐	☐	☐	☐	☐
22. Unmarried expectant teen	☐	☐	☐	☐	☐
27. Alcoholic	☐	☐	☐	☐	☐
Religious					
3. Jew	☐	☐	☐	☐	☐
8. Catholic	☐	☐	☐	☐	☐
13. Jehovah's Witness	☐	☐	☐	☐	☐
18. Atheist	☐	☐	☐	☐	☐
23. Protestant	☐	☐	☐	☐	☐
28. Amish	☐	☐	☐	☐	☐

(continues)

Level of Response Individual	1 Greet	2 Accept	3 Help	4 Background	5 Advocate
Physically/Mentally challenged					
4. Person with Hemophilia	☐	☐	☐	☐	☐
9. Senile elderly person	☐	☐	☐	☐	☐
14. Cerebral palsied person	☐	☐	☐	☐	☐
19. Person with AIDS	☐	☐	☐	☐	☐
24. Amputee	☐	☐	☐	☐	☐
29. Person with cancer	☐	☐	☐	☐	☐
Political					
5. Neo-Nazi	☐	☐	☐	☐	☐
10. Teamster Union member	☐	☐	☐	☐	☐
15. E.R.A. proponent	☐	☐	☐	☐	☐
20. Communist	☐	☐	☐	☐	☐
25. Ku Klux Klansman	☐	☐	☐	☐	☐
30. Nuclear armament proponent	☐	☐	☐	☐	☐

Exercise Three: Assessing Your Personal Responses to Transcultural Health Care Situations

When asked to care for a client from a different cultural background, it is natural to have some concerns. How do you feel about working with clients who are from a very different culture than your own, or who do not speak English? Are you worried that you will not be able to communicate clearly with these clients? Try to respond as honestly as possible to the statements below.

	Agree	Neutral	Disagree
People are the same. I don't behave any differently toward people from a cultural background that differs from mine.	____	____	____
I always know what to say to someone from a different cultural background.	____	____	____
I look forward to caring for a client from a different cultural background.	____	____	____
I know how to care for a client who does not speak any English.	____	____	____
I can learn something when I care for clients from diverse cultural backgrounds.	____	____	____
I always introduce myself to the client's family.	____	____	____
I prefer to care for a client from my own cultural group who speaks my language because it is easier.	____	____	____

Exercise Four: Examining Your Cultural Values

This exercise is designed to help you explore your cultural values (which are most likely Western) in relationship to the cultural values of non-Western cultural groups. This exercise contains nine pairs of statements that have relevance to health care. The statements on the left represent Western values, whereas the statements on the right represent values held elsewhere in the world. As you rate each statement, *try to be as truthful with yourself as possible*. If you are really honest, you may be surprised at how many of your answers are heavily biased toward Western values.

CULTURAL VALUES

Directions

Circle 1—If you strongly agree with the statement on the left.
Circle 2—If you agree with the statement on the left.
Circle 3—If you agree with the statement on the right.
Circle 4—If you strongly agree with the statement on the right.

1. Responsible adults prepare for the future and strive to influence events in their lives.	1 2 3 4	Life follows a preordained course. The outcome of events is beyond our control.
2. It is confusing and dishonest to give vague and tentative answers.	1 2 3 4	It is best to avoid direct and honest answers because you may offend and embarrass others.
3. Intelligent, efficient people use their time well and are always punctual.	1 2 3 4	Being punctual to work or a meeting is not as important as enjoying relaxed and pleasant times with family and friends.
4. Stoicism is the appropriate response to severe pain.	1 2 3 4	Loudly crying out and moaning is an appropriate response to severe pain.
5. It is not wise to accept a gift from a person you do not know.	1 2 3 4	It is important to accept gifts and thus avoid insulting the giver.
6. It is a sign of friendliness to address people by their first names.	1 2 3 4	It is disrespectful to address people by their first names unless they give you permission to do so.
7. The best way to gain information is to ask direct questions.	1 2 3 4	It is rude and intrusive to obtain information by asking direct questions.
8. Direct eye contact shows that you are an honest person and that you are interested in the other person.	1 2 3 4	Avoiding direct eye contact may imply that you are not being honest, or you are not interested in what the other person is saying.
9. Ultimately, the needs of the individual are more important than the needs of the family.	1 2 3 4	The needs of the family far outweigh the needs of the individual.

Adapted from Renwick, G.W. & Rhinesmith, S.H. *An Exercise in Cultural Analysis for Managers.* Chicago, Intercultural Press, Inc. Published in: Thiederman, S.B. Ethnocentrism: A barrier to effective health care. *Nurse Practitioner.* 11(8):52–59, 1986.

Exercise Five: Setting Up Your *Transcultural Interaction Diary*

Perhaps at some time you have kept a diary or a journal for recording your thoughts, feelings, activities, and memorable events. To improve your transcultural communication, you need to set up and keep a *Transcultural Interaction Diary*. This diary will provide you with a record of your experiences with clients and other health care professionals from different cultures. You can use your diary to (1) record your transcultural verbal and non-verbal communications; (2) analyze your feelings concerning these transactions, (3) plan strategies for improving your transcultural communications, and (4) record the outcomes from these strategies.

To set up your *Transcultural Interaction Diary*, follow these simple steps:

1. Decide on a "form" for your diary. For example, you can use legal pads, spiral note books, note cards, "locked" diaries, empty books, or computer discs.

2. Keep your diary in a private place. You will not feel as free to write about negative interactions or feelings if you think other people will read your material.

3. Write in your diary on a regular basis—preferably every time that you have a significant (very positive or negative) transcultural interaction. It is important to record conversations, thoughts, and feelings while they are still fresh in your memory.

4. Start to write in your diary *now*, before reading the chapters in this unit. Think back and record any significant transcultural interactions that you had before you entered health care, and since you have been in health care. Be sure to write down both verbal and nonverbal communications, as well as the thoughts and feelings that you had during and after each interaction.

5. As you study Unit 1, write down any *new* transcultural interactions in your diary. Note how you are using the information in each chapter to increase your ability to communicate with the different cultural groups within your health care subculture.

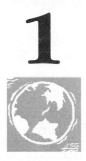

CHAPTER

1

INTRODUCTION TO TRANSCULTURAL COMMUNICATION IN HEALTH CARE

Margaret A. McKenna

KEY TERMS

- Body Language
- Communication Competence
- Cultural Diversity
- Dyad
- Exchange Process
- Oral Language
- Population Categories

OBJECTIVES

After completing this chapter, you should be able to:

- Begin to interact with individuals in an exchange–negotiation process.
- Describe the dimensions of communication competence.
- List and explain the four reasons transcultural communication is urgently needed in the health care workplace today.
- Discuss the danger of relying on the statistical categories developed by the United States government for categorizing people into five population groups.

11

INTRODUCTION

The delivery of health care depends on clear communication between the individuals who are involved—for example clients, physicians, health care professionals, interpreters, and family members. Clear communication is essential in any health care context, be it a physician's office, an acute care unit, a client's home, an extended care facility, dental office, or other health care setting.

The most common form of communication is the **dyad** or interaction between two people. The dyad of a health care professional and a client is the primary form of interaction in most health care settings. Health care professionals may also speak to groups of people, and they may teach clients with similar needs in a classroom setting. An example is a diabetes class. But most often, the health care professional communicates with one client at a time, with the goal of making that exchange as effective, appropriate, and acceptable to both parties as possible.

Unfortunately, any communication between health care professional and client can be reduced in quality and marked by frustration. Frustration arises when the health care professional gives too little attention to the cultural background of the client and its influence on communication. This text focuses on how to improve the quality of transcultural communication between clients and health care professionals and between health care professionals and other staff members. To improve your interactions with people from diverse backgrounds, you will need to learn more about different cultures and develop your communication skills.

COMMUNICATION: A CORNERSTONE
FOR HEALTH CARE PRACTICE

To successfully work with clients from other cultures, you must continually strive for clear communication and mutual understanding. In many interactions, communication is cloudy because health care professionals incorrectly assume that their clients understand what they are trying to communicate.

COMMUNICATION CONSIDERATIONS

 To improve your interaction with clients from other cultures, you should assess the client's level of understanding rather than assume that a client understands what you are saying.

One way to improve transcultural communication effectiveness is to think of your interaction with a client as an **exchange process**, not as a one-sided provider-to-client path of information. A satisfactory health care interaction between a provider and a client is really one of exchange and negotiation.

Consider this exchange process as a scale that can be weighted in favor of one side or that can be balanced between your proposed plan of care and your client's beliefs and preferences for care. For example, your client may believe strongly in complimentary (alternative) therapies. If that is the case, you could ignore the client's interest in complimentary therapies, a strategy that would probably upset the client. Or you could take the client's beliefs into consideration as you develop your plan of care.

In an exchange with a client from another culture, you need to know:

1. How and when to start a conversation.
2. How best to be understood; for example, you may need an interpreter.
3. How to respond to a client's gestures or questions.
4. How to be sensitive to the client's reactions.
5. How to listen to the client's concerns.
6. How to take the client's illness and health-related beliefs into consideration as you plan care.

These dimensions are the basis for **communication competence**. The primary objective of this textbook is to bring you closer to transcultural communication competence. To improve your transcultural communication skills, read each chapter carefully and work through the self-assessment and self-evaluation exercises that are at the beginning and end of each Unit. You can also develop competence in transcultural communication by following these steps:

- Assess your own cultural background.
- Identify the values that underlie your behavior.
- Recognize that communication is influenced and determined by your culture.
- Recognize that there are many cultures that interact in a health care setting.

LANGUAGE AND COMMUNICATION

Language is the primary means used by humans to communicate with each other. Humans have developed written, sign, and oral languages in order to share messages. Humans use language to express ideas, feelings, and emotions; to communicate information, reactions, and directions to each other; and to negotiate with each other.

Oral language is a feature of every society. In a health care setting, oral language is used to verbally communicate with clients and other health care professionals. Caregivers need to recognize that individuals also communicate in nonverbal ways.

People communicate with **body language**, a topic that is discussed in greater detail in Chapter 3. Sign language, a form of body language, is the native language of members of deaf communities. It is important to remember that there are many cross-cultural similarities in body language, but there are also key differences. The meaning of different gestures varies from culture to culture. Never assume that a gesture holds the same meaning for you and your client—especially if your client is from another culture.

As you work with clients, you will encounter a great diversity in spoken languages. For instance, over 6000 languages and dialects are spoken today. Mandarin Chinese is spoken by 836 million people. In the late 1990s, there are nearly as many Spanish speakers (who number 332 million) as there are Hindi speakers (who number 333 million worldwide) (Microsoft Encarta 97 Encyclopedia, 1996). There are 322 million English speakers. If we were to include individuals who speak English as a second language (with Mandarin Chinese being the most widely spoken), then English is the second most widely spoken language, with 418 million speakers.

Although you cannot expect to be familiar with even a portion of these languages, you can still find ways to communicate with clients who do not speak or understand English. In Chapter 9, you will find helpful suggestions on how to communicate clearly with clients who are not proficient in English, with or without an interpreter.

THE GROWING DEMAND FOR TRANSCULTURAL COMMUNICATION

There are mounting reasons for health care professionals to become competent in transcultural communication. The motivating forces that provide the momentum for implementing transcultural communication come from several sources:

1. There is increasing ethnic, racial, and **cultural diversity** in the composition of the United States population.

2. Clients represent many cultural, ethnic, and disenfranchised populations, and they have different culturally influenced patterns of behavior and expectations for care. Moreover, clients are increasingly more diverse in heritage, experiences, and lifestyle.

3. Settings for health care delivery are multicultural and multinational.

4. Health care professions have a commitment to provide high quality, culturally appropriate care.

Increasing Diversity in Population Composition

The ethnic and racial composition of the population of the United States has been changing dramatically for the past decade. There is increasing diversity in languages, beliefs, lifestyles, and practices among residents in rural and urban areas throughout the country. The percentage of the United States population that is white has decreased since the 1970s. This reduction in population is due in part to increasing immigration from Asia and Latin American nations, and in part due to a higher population growth rate among blacks.

Based on the 1990 census, the black population in the United States has grown by more than 14% between 1980 and 1990. The percent of persons of Hispanic origin increased 53% from 1980 to 1990 (American Heritage Concise Dictionary, 1994). These statistics will be updated in the 2000 census. Asians and Pacific Islanders in the United States now number 7.5 million—a figure that has doubled from 1980 when this ethnic group numbered 3.7 million. This increase in the population of ethnic groups means that health care services will have to address the needs of clients from diverse cultural, ethnic, and racial backgrounds.

Multicultural Client Groups

It is not unusual to hear a number of languages and dialects spoken among clients in a large medical center, especially in an urban or suburban setting. In a northwestern city in the United States, each of the hospitals, clinics, and other health care settings may care for families who speak as many as 40 different languages.

Health care professionals will continue to encounter clients in many different health care settings who speak a language other than English. In the United States, nearly 32 million residents who are 5 years or older speak a language other than English at home (Microsoft Encarta 97 Encyclopedia, 1996). The majority of that number (54%) speak Spanish. The other languages most frequently spoken in the United States are Chinese, Tagalog, Polish, Korean, Vietnamese, Portuguese, Japanese, Greek, Arabic, Hindi and Urdu, Russian, Yiddish, Thai, Lao, Persian, French, Creole, Armenian, and Navaho (Microsoft Encarta 97 Encyclopedia, 1996).

Multinational and Multicultural Workplaces

Health care professionals practice in a multicultural environment, even if they think of themselves as belonging to one culture or as "just being American." The misunderstandings that develop in health care settings may occur between providers, as well as between clients and providers from different cultural backgrounds. Many health care professionals would find these words familiar: "I can't understand why this family won't do what I ask," or "I hope I don't have to work with that individual again. I'm never sure he understands what I am talking about."

Two goals of this book are to (1) discuss the barriers that can block transcultural communication among health care professionals, and (2) provide clear guidelines for recognizing and overcoming these barriers in the workplace.

COMMUNICATION CONSIDERATIONS

To work effectively as team members and provide safe client care, health care professionals must commit to increasing communication in the workplace, particularly when team members are from diverse cultures.

All health care professionals need to commit themselves to enhancing their knowledge of different cultures and developing their skills in transcultural communication. You can gain a knowledge of different cultures by reading about cultures, seeing films about different cultures, talking with clients or co-workers about their cultural backgrounds, or acting as a participant-observer in a cultural setting such as an ethnic neighborhood. You can develop transcultural communication skills by first assessing your level of skill, practicing various techniques to improve your skills, evaluating your new skills, and deciding what improvements you still need to make.

COMMUNICATION CONSIDERATIONS

Improving your transcultural communication with clients and team members is an on-going process. Every new person you meet who is from another culture will help to broaden your appreciation of different cultures and improve your transcultural communication skills.

VITAL REMARKS AND SPECIAL CAUTIONS

For the purpose of collecting statistics, the United States and Canadian governments have categorized people into five general **population categories**: white, black, Hispanic, Asian, and Native American. These categories are used in health care settings as well as in schools, government facilities, and businesses. Unfortunately, the use of these five categories has tended to diminish the very essence of quality health care. That is, the widespread use of such broad categories has blurred or even extinguished the crucial cultural differences between the individuals and the groups within each population census category (Andrews & Boyle, 1998).

COMMUNICATION CONSIDERATIONS

People should not be stereotyped simply because they are members of a broad, statistically defined, racial or ethnic category. Although clients and health care professionals may share values with other people from their race or culture, they are first and foremost individuals.

It is important to recognize that within each of the broad, statistical categories there are numerous cultural groups. These groups are characterized by variations in lifestyle, values and beliefs, health- and illness-related practices, preferences for care, and family member patterns of interaction. For example, there are many cultural groups that are included in the category of *white* (sometimes also referred to as Anglo-American or Caucasian). Individuals in these groups may trace their heritage to a European nation, Australia, North America, or many other nations and regions. Among individuals who are white, the largest group of 58 million people have a German ancestry. Another 38.7 million Americans trace their roots to Ireland, and more than 32 million Americans have an English ancestry (1990 United States Census).

There is also great diversity among the individuals who are included in the *Hispanic* population category. There are differences in their countries of origin, in the dialects spoken, and in customs and beliefs including practices related to health and illness. For example, among Spanish speakers, there are many variations in the use of words and expressions. Clients from different states in Mexico have different dialects, and they do not necessarily understand individuals from Puerto Rico or Cuba. Recent immigrants from Mexico may speak an Indian dialect or a mixture of Spanish and Mixtec.

The term *black* is similarly very inclusive, and may refer to individuals who are recent refugees or immigrants from African nations or individuals who can trace their heritage through multiple generations of residence in the United States. Furthermore, the term *Native American* too often blurs the distinctions among members of more than 500 Native American nations who reside in North America. Likewise, the term *Asian* refers to the Japanese, Chinese, Indochinese, Filipino, Korean, Vietnamese, and Indian populations, each of which contains numerous, diverse subcultures.

In this book, the five population census categories are presented. However, we emphasize that each of these categories contain many different cultural groups which, in turn, are comprised of people with their own individual ideas, beliefs, and values. Each chapter contains examples and brief clinical interactions that illustrate how to use transcultural communication skills to interact with clients from a variety of cultural backgrounds. Chapter 13 also describes skills for interacting with staff members from diverse backgrounds.

COMMUNICATION CONSIDERATIONS

Always consider clients and co-workers from other cultures as **individuals** *with unique experiences and expectations, and then as members of different cultures.*

TESTING YOUR KNOWLEDGE

Circle the correct answer.

1. The primary form of communication is called the
   a. interchange.
   b. dyad.
   c. doublet.
   d. deuce.

2. Language involves
   a. oral speech.
   b. gestures.
   c. signing.
   d. all of the above.

3. From the 1970s to the 1990s, the percentage of the United States population that is white has
   a. increased.
   b. decreased.
   c. stayed the same.
   d. shifted from the suburbs into the cities.

4. Since 1980, the black population of the United States has
   a. increased.
   b. decreased.
   c. stayed the same.
   d. shifted from the suburbs into the cities.

5. The number of people in the United States 5 years or older that speak a language other than English is around
   a. 10 million people.
   b. 20 million people.
   c. 30 million people.
   d. 50 million people.

2

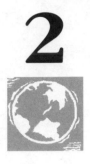

TRANSCULTURAL COMMUNICATION BUILDING BLOCKS: CULTURE AND CULTURAL VALUES

KEY TERMS

- African American
- Amor Propio
- Ashkenazi Jews
- Asian
- Black
- Conservative Jews
- Cultural Values
- Culture
- Culture Shock
- Deitsch
- Demut
- Filipino
- Gelassenheit
- Galang
- Hasidic Jews
- Hispanic
- Holocaust
- Kosher
- Lace Curtain Irish

- Latino
- Monotheistic
- Muslim
- Native American
- Old Order Amish
- Orthodox Jews
- Pilipino
- Pogroms
- Reform Jews
- Sabras
- Sephardic Jews
- Shanty Irish
- Subculture
- Tagalog
- Torah
- Treyf
- Tzedakah
- WASP
- Zerangi

OBJECTIVES

After completing this chapter, you should be able to:

- Define *culture* and discuss its role in determining the philosophy and values of individuals and groups.

- Define *subculture* and describe the different subcultures that are a part of American culture.

- Define *cultural values* and provide at least 7 reasons that values are so important.

- Differentiate between the major value systems of different cultural groups.

- Acquire information about the beliefs and values of the specific cultural groups with whom you routinely work.

INTRODUCTION

Transcultural communication involves the successful interchange of ideas and feelings between people from different cultures. For health care professionals, the ability to communicate transculturally with clients and their families often spells the difference between success and frustration when assessing clients and providing their care. The study of culture provides the foundation necessary for understanding and fostering transcultural communication. This chapter discusses the meaning of culture and explores the ways in which culture affects a person's values, beliefs, behavior, and communication style.

CULTURE

Culture refers to the common lifestyles, languages, behavior patterns, traditions, and beliefs that are learned and passed from one generation to the next. Culture helps to determine a person's world view or philosophy of life, and it influences how each of us views our relationship to our surrounding environment, religion, time, and each other. Culture provides each person with specific rules for dealing with the universal events of life—birth, mating, child-rearing, illness, pain, and death.

Although culture provides strength and stability, it is never static. Cultural groups face continual challenges from such powerful forces as environmental upheavals, plagues, wars, migrations, the influx of immigrants, and the growth of new technologies. As a result, cultures change and evolve over time.

Culture is learned and then shared. People learn about their culture from parents, teachers, religious and political leaders, and respected peers. As children grow up, they gradually internalize the values and beliefs of their culture, and they, in turn, share these values and beliefs with their children.

Normally, children learn about their culture while growing up. However, when people migrate from their native culture into a new culture, they often experience **culture shock**. Culture shock develops when the values and beliefs upheld by this new culture are radically different from the person's native culture. For successful assimilation into a new culture, immigrants must learn and internalize that culture's important values.

In addition to belonging to a major cultural group, people also belong to a variety of **subcultures** or smaller groups within a culture. Each subculture has its own value system and related expectations for behavior. Subcultures may be based on:

1. Professional and occupational affiliations (American Medical Association, American Nurses Association)

2. Nationality or race (a shared historical and political past)

3. Age groups (adolescents, senior citizens)

4. Gender (feminists, mens' groups)

5. Socioeconomic factors (the working class, the middle class, the upper class)

6. Political viewpoints (Democrat, Republican)

For example, when you began your study of health care, you entered a subculture, and initially you probably suffered from some degree of culture shock. You had to learn a whole new value system. During your years of study, you gradually internalized the values taught by your instructors. Eventually you became comfortable with the values and behaviors you learned and by the time you graduated, you had been assimilated into the professional health care subculture.

Upon entering a health care setting, clients also become members of a subculture. In this world filled with strange sights, unfamiliar sounds, and strangers, many clients experience culture shock. This shock intensifies for clients who are recent immigrants or who do not speak English.

COMMUNICATION CONSIDERATIONS

Because health care professionals and clients belong to different subcultures, their interaction is always to some extent transcultural, even when the health care professional and client come from the same general culture.

In summary, culture has a powerful impact on individuals, groups, and entire societies, influencing all aspects of human life. Cultures and subcultures provide strategies and methods for coping with life's ever-changing challenges and demands. Family, childrearing, economics, education, health beliefs, and healthcare are all dramatically influenced by culture and the values and beliefs that it engenders.

CULTURAL VALUES

Cultural values are principles or standards that members of a cultural group share in common. Values dramatically differ from culture to culture. People educated in mainstream, white, American, middle-class culture may have very different values from people raised in the many and varied Asian, Hispanic, black, or Native American cultures. Accepting and respecting the values of clients from other cultures is the first step toward successful transcultural communication.

Values serve several important functions:

1. They provide people with a set of rules by which to govern their lives.
2. They serve as a basis for attitudes, beliefs, and behaviors.
3. They help to guide actions and decisions.
4. They give direction to people's lives and help them solve common problems.
5. They influence how individuals perceive and react to other individuals.
6. They help determine basic attitudes regarding personal, social, and philosophical issues.
7. They reflect a person's identity and provide a basis for self-evaluation.

VALUES OF MAJOR AMERICAN CULTURAL GROUPS

The following general guidelines compare and contrast the basic traditional values of the five major cultural groups that are predominant in American Society: white, Asian, Hispanic, black, and Native American. However, it is vital to recognize that many individuals do not follow their culture's traditional values because they have either assimilated the values of a different culture, or because they have formulated their own value system. Although these guidelines will help you to understand a client's general cultural background, some of your clients may believe in values that are different from those traditionally accepted in their cultures.

COMMUNICATION CONSIDERATIONS

 Remember that each person is first and foremost an individual, and secondly a member of a cultural group.

White Values

The prevailing value system for many white Americans is primarily based on the white, Anglo-Saxon, Protestant (**WASP**) ethic (Sue & Sue, 1999). This ethic traces its origins to the white Protestants who came to this country from Northern Europe over two centuries ago. Values that still dominate the white American middle-class ethic include independence, individuality, wealth, comfort, cleanliness, achievement, punctuality, hard work, aggression, assertiveness, rationality, an orientation toward the future, and mastery of one's own fate (Andrews & Boyle, 1998; Edmission, 1997).

Traditionally, most white Americans have wanted to be recognized as *individuals* rather than as members of groups. Thus white Americans, unlike members of many other cultures, tend to be competitive with each other rather than cooperative. White American culture also values the nuclear family and its traditions.

COMMUNICATION CONSIDERATIONS

 Many white Americans do not belong to the mainstream culture, but instead belong to ethnic subcultures that hold strong values of their own (e.g., Irish, Jewish, Iranian, German, Italian, Norwegian, Appalachian, and Amish subcultures).

Asian Values

Within the United States, **Asian** (or *Asian American*) is a term that primarily encompasses the Japanese, Chinese, Indochinese, Filipino, Korean, Vietnamese, and Indian populations. These populations are highly diverse; indeed, members of these groups speak different languages and encounter different life experiences. The Asian-American population is growing rapidly. Based on the 1990 census, the annual rate of growth of the Asian-American population is estimated at 4%. In 1990, there were 7.5 million Asians within the United States, and that population may increase to 17 million by the year 2010 (American Diversity, 1991). These statistics will be updated in the 2000 census.

Traditional Asian values are firmly rooted in traditional religious beliefs. Chinese, Vietnamese, and Korean values have been greatly influenced by Buddhism, Taoism, Christianity, and Confucianism (Compton's, 1995).

- *Buddhism* is a doctrine that is attributed to Siddhartha Gautama, the *Buddha* or *The Enlightened One*. Buddha lived around 2500 years ago in India. Buddhism teaches that suffering is an inevitable part of life. Devout Buddhists believe that by extinguishing their sense of self and their desires, they can pass beyond suffering into a state of perfect illumination or enlightenment, called Nirvana. One-eighth of the world's population believes in Buddhism.

- *Taoism,* another Eastern philosophy and religion, is based on the teachings of Lao-tse who lived in China during the 6th century BC. The word *Tao* means *way,* suggesting a way of thinking and living. Like the God of the Christians and Jews, Tao is viewed as the essential unifying element of all that is. Taoism teaches that a person should cultivate a mystical relationship to the Tao, shun worldly desires, and avoid lusting after wealth and power. For a Taoist, the most important goal is to live an orderly life that is in harmony with the universe.

- *Christianity* is based on the teachings of Jesus of Nazareth, who was born in Bethlehem of Judea. More than 1 billion people throughout the world believe in the teachings of Jesus Christ. Christianity is split into many different groups, the three largest being the Roman Catholic Church, Eastern Orthodox Churches, and Protestant Churches. Although different churches have their own interpretation of Christian doctrine, all churches agree that the ideal Christian is compassionate, kind, humble, gentle, patient, and forgiving.

- *Confucianism* was founded by the great teacher Confucius, who lived from 551 to 479 BC. Because of his teachings and wise sayings (which are similar to the proverbs in the Bible), Confucius was revered in China almost like a God. Temples erected to honor Confucius were built in most of the major cities in China. Although Confucianism is considered a religion, it is actually a moral code of conduct. Confucius encouraged his followers to live a virtuous life filled with goodness and kind deeds. Confucius also taught that it was important to be accountable to one's family and neighbors, and that elders and well-educated people deserve special consideration and respect.

Japanese religious values are primarily based on Zen Buddhism and Shintoism, whereas the religious beliefs of East Indians evolved from Hinduism.

• *Zen Buddhism* is a form of Buddhism that was transplanted from China to Japan around the 12th century AD. Zen is a Japanese term meaning *meditation*. Zen Buddhism was the religion of the Samurai warriors during the 14th and 15th centuries, and it dominated Japanese culture during the 16th century. In the 1950s, Alan Watts, a British philosopher, introduced Americans to Zen Buddhism through his book *The Way of Zen*. Zen Buddhism teaches that there is only one reality, and that this reality can be understood only through meditation and intuition, not reason and analysis. Devout followers of Zen may seek to enter a monastery where they and their masters can find enlightenment through a life devoted to service, prayer, and meditation (Compton, 1995).

• *Shintoism, way of the gods* or *kami way*, is the indigenous religion of Japan. Ancient Shintoism arose from a belief in kami which means god or gods, above, superior, or divine. Shintoists believe that because kami manifests itself in nature (mountains, trees, birds, rivers, and stars) and in human beings, the entire universe is bound together by kami. Today there are over 80,000 Shinto shrines throughout the world. Like their ancient predecessors, modern Shintoists strive to embrace kami in their daily lives by performing various rituals and by participating in Shinto festivals and holidays. Present-day Shintoists may also petition their deities for material blessings such as a new car or home (Zich, 1991; Zehavi, 1973).

• *Hinduism* is the major religion of the Indian subcontinent. The word Hindu is derived from an ancient Sanskrit term and means dwellers by the Indus River. The dwellers are the people who developed the Indus Valley Civilization almost 4000 years ago. Hinduism has no founder and no specific doctrine. Whereas Hinduism is characterized by a great diversity of beliefs, most Hindus adhere to the following religious tenets:

1. there is only one God called Brahman

2. all forms of nature and life are sacred

3. individuals pass through many cycles of life and death (transmigration of souls) and they may be reincarnated as human beings, animals, or even plants

4. the priesthood is hereditary, and individuals may become priests only through reincarnation

5. the way an individual lives in this life determines the next life (the doctrine of Karman or law of cause and effect).

Today, 90% of Hindus live in India, and the remaining 10% dwell in South Africa, Trinidad, Europe, and the United States (Miller & Goodin, 1995; Compton, 1995).

Traditional Asian values and mainstream American values may differ in several ways. Whereas Western culture values independence and self-reliance, many Asian cultures place a higher value on subordination of personal interests to those of the family. For instance, some Asian family members will likely put aside their own work, needs, and interests to care for a sick or elderly relative. Also Asians usually have a strong group orientation which extends to the workplace.

Example: Some Asian health care professionals may accept assignments without complaint that mainstream American health care professionals might resent. This is because Asian individuals are more likely to value the *combined work* of the health care team over the work of an individual member. Additionally, an Asian health care professional may feel that it is inappropriate for a subordinate to challenge a supervisor. American workers who feel unfairly treated are more likely to complain to their supervisors than Asian workers.

Table 2-1 identifies traditional Asian values and representative mainstream American values. Remember however, that individuals may hold some traditional Asian values and some mainstream American values. For example, a person might value older people and the past, but also value young people and the future, which could create a conflict when values clash. Another person's values may lie somewhere between traditional Asian and mainstream American values.

Hispanic Values

Hispanic is a broad term that refers to

1. groups with cultural and national identities arising from the Caribbean, Mexico, and Central and South America and

2. individuals who trace their ancestry to Spain and identify themselves as Hispanic.

Thus, the term *Hispanic* is not linked to race but rather to culture and nationality. The use of Hispanic is generally preferred to *Chicano*. The word **Latino** is sometimes used as an alternative to Hispanic. Many prefer Latino because

Table 2-1	
Examples of Traditional Asian Values and Mainstream American Values	
Asian Values	**American Values**
Group orientation	Independence, self-reliance, and individualism
Submission to authority	Resistance to authority
Extended family	Nuclear/blended family
Tradition	Innovation
Respect for elders	Emphasis on youth
Respect for the past	Future oriented
Conformity	Competition

it implies cultural ties to South America rather than Spain (Barnhart & Metcalf, 1997). According to the 1990 census, in 1990, there were 22.5 million people of Hispanic origin in the United States. The Hispanic population is expected to grow to 40.5 million by 2000 (American Diversity, 1991). These statistics will be updated in the 2000 census. In addition, the Census Bureau reports that by 2005, Hispanics will be the nation's largest minority group, outnumbering blacks, who are currently the leading minority (Holmes, 1998).

The Hispanics—including Mexican-Americans, Cubans, Salvadorans, Guatemalans, Puerto Ricans, and others—greatly value the family, and often place the needs of family members above the needs of individuals. Family members are typically respectful and affectionate toward one another. The extended family may include not only blood relatives, but non-blood relatives such as godparents.

Many Hispanics value the development and nurturing of close interpersonal relationships. When a Hispanic family member is ill, family members usually give their sick relative abundant physical and emotional support. Because family ties are so valued, Hispanic clients usually want extended family members present during a hospitalization. Also, some Hispanic family members prefer to be involved in the decisions pertaining to their loved one's care.

In addition to valuing the family, many Hispanics have traditionally valued religion, especially Catholicism and the celebration of the Catholic Mass. Because of a deep religious faith, many Hispanics believe in self-sacrifice, giving rather than taking, enduring hardships, and acceptance of fate. Finally, Hispanics typically value the present over the future. Most Hispanics feel that enjoying leisure activities with family members is as important as working.

Table 2-2

Examples of Traditional Hispanic and Mainstream American Values

Hispanic Values	American Values
Group emphasis	Individuality
Extended family	Nuclear/blended family
Person-to-person orientation	Person-to-object orientation
Acceptance/resignation	Aggression/assertion
Fatalistic	Master of one's own fate
Present oriented	Future oriented

Table 2-2 summarizes some common differences in values between Hispanic culture and mainstream American culture. Remember as with Table 2-1, individuals may not subscribe to every value held by a group. Some individuals may hold both traditional Hispanic values and mainstream American values. A person's values can also be influenced by occupation, level of education, income and work status, as well as the values of family or significant others.

Black Values

The term **black**, like the terms *Hispanic* or *Asian*, erroneously lumps together a highly diverse group of people who came to the United States from many parts of the world. According to the 1990 census, blacks are currently the largest minority group in the United States, numbering approximately 30.6 million (12.3% of the population) in 1990. The black population is expected to expand to 40.2 million (13.4% of the population) by 2010 (American Diversity, 1991). These statistics will be updated in the 2000 census.

Although the largest group of blacks is of African descent, some Blacks trace their recent ancestry—and consequently their cultural identity—to nations in the Caribbean. In some areas, blacks refer to themselves as Eritreans, Kenyans, African Americans, Haitians, or Dominicans (from the Dominican Republic).

Terms for black Americans have evolved over the 20th century from *colored* to *Negro* to *black*, to *Afro-American*, to **African American**, a term that became popular after it was used in 1988 by Jesse Jackson. Many black Americans prefer the term *African American* to black because of its emphasis on heritage rather than color (Barnhart & Metcalf, 1997). However, the name

African American does not encompass the thousands of black Americans whose recent ancestry is from areas other than Africa, such as the Caribbean.

Some black Americans do have different values from what we refer to as mainstream white American values. Unlike mainstream white Americans, however, many blacks experienced and struggled against racism perpetuated by both white individuals and institutions. In some ways, many blacks have adopted values that reflect their experiences in an environment dominated by white culture. Because of a perceived need for solidarity, some blacks seek the solace and strength that lie in the family, church, and black community.

Blacks traditionally have been more present-oriented than whites. Some blacks still focus on the present because they believe the future will contain the same elements of racism and discrimination that oppressed them in the past. Other blacks actively plan for the future and strive for higher education and professional status.

Although many of us have a stereotyped view of a dominant female figure as the head of black households, a woman's role varies depending on the family. In some families, the mother, grandmother, or aunt is the primary caretaker of several children; however, families vary in their composition and in the roles assumed by family members.

Table 2-3 summarizes some common differences in the traditional values of black and white American cultures. As you review Table 2-3, remember that individuals may or may not choose to follow the traditional values of their culture. Also, people who belong to different cultures but share similar educational, economic, and occupational backgrounds will likely share similar values. For example, blacks and whites who graduate from a university and pursue professional careers may also share similar values concerning financial security, family, childrearing, and education.

Table 2-3

Examples of Values of Blacks Primarily from Black Communities and Mainstream White American Values

Values Common to Blacks	Values Common to Mainstream Whites
Family bonding	Individualism
Matrifocal	Patrifocal
Present oriented	Future oriented
Spiritual orientation	Personal mastery

Native American Values

Native Americans (American Indians) are a highly heterogeneous group that includes approximately 530 different tribal groups. According to the 1990 U.S. Census and the Source Book of Zip Code Demographics, the 5 largest Native American communities or cultural nations in the lower 48 states are:

1. Cherokee, 308,132 people

2. Navajo, 219,198 people

3. Chippewa, 103,826 people

4. Sioux, 103,255 people

5. Choctaw, 81,299 people

Although the U.S. Census scheduled for the year 2000 may prove differently, the 1990 U.S. Census also reported that the Native American population of Alaska is composed of:

- 21,869 American Indian/Athapaskan people who live in both Alaska and Canada

- 10,052 Aleuts who inhabit the Aleutian Islands and the Alaskan peninsula

- 44,400 Eskimos who primarily live near the Bering Sea and the Arctic Ocean coasts (Lefever & Davidhizar, 1999)

Most Native Americans are burdened with poverty. For example, on the Navajo reservation, only 60% of homes have adequate plumbing, a bedroom, or are hooked to a public sewer system; only 23% of homes have a telephone; only 6% use electricity for heat. Typically, wood serves as the major heating fuel for a reservation home (1990 U.S. Census).

According to the U.S. Department of Housing and Urban Development–U.S. Census Bureau, 30% of Native Americans live below the poverty line, compared with 29.5% of blacks, 25.3% of Hispanics, 14.1% of Asian/Pacific Islanders, and 9.8% of whites. Also, Native Americans have the lowest life expectancy of any ethnic group in the United States. Native Americans can expect to live only two-thirds as long as other people in the United States.

Many Native American families take pride in maintaining a traditional lifestyle and prefer the ways of their grandparents. They may not want to embrace all of the values of the mainstream American culture. There are many variations in family patterns of blending mainstream values and urban ways, with traditional values and what some term *Indian ways*.

Traditional culture can give individual Native Americans security and a sense of belonging. Members who decide to leave the reservation to pursue opportunities in the broader world outside may suffer from a loss of identity, as traditional values clash with new lifestyles.

Example: When a white, middle-class youth decides to go away to college, proud parents may view this action as a welcome sign that their child is ambitious and goal-oriented. When a Native American youth leaves the reservation to seek a college education, elders may interpret this action in many ways: the youth may be relinquishing identity with family and community members, acquiring different values, or preparing to help or care for other Native Americans.

Many Native Americans value the extended family. Thus grandparents, aunts, and uncles—even though they live in separate households—are actively involved in raising the children. Women play a major role in working with and educating youth.

Other Native American values include:

- The importance of sharing one's worldly goods with others rather than hoarding possessions

- Cooperating with others, rather than competing against others

- Working for the good of the group, rather than the good of the individual

- Respecting the rights of others, rather than interfering with others

- Being involved with the present rather than the future

- Accepting nature and the natural order of things, rather than trying to control nature

Table 2-4 summarizes some differences in the traditional values of Native Americans and mainstream white Americans.

VALUES OF OTHER SELECTED AMERICAN CULTURAL GROUPS

Although the five broad cultural groups just discussed have had an enormous impact on American values, there are many other important cultural groups that have immigrated to the new world, bringing their values with them. Indeed, the United States is a land that has been built, in large part, by immigrants. Since the early 1700s, hundreds of thousands of immigrants fleeing from poverty, war, and religious persecution have come to this nation in search of wealth and freedom. Immigrants have come from all over the world— Europe, the British Isles, the Middle East, Asia, India, and the Philippines—

Table 2-4

Examples of Values of Native Americans Who Primarily Live on Reservations and Mainstream White Americans

Values Common to Some Native Americans	Values Common To Some Mainstream Whites
Bonding to family or group	Individualism
Sharing with others	Accumulating for self
Present oriented	Future oriented
Extended family	Nuclear family
Cooperation	Competition
Acceptance of nature	Mastery over nature

to help build the American way of life. Due to space limitations, this section discusses the values of five of the many vital cultures that have settled in the United States: the Amish, Filipinos, Iranians, Irish, and Jews.

Amish Values

The **Old Order Amish** (pronounced ah-mish) is an ethnoreligious group that migrated from Germany to the United States almost 300 years ago. Like other groups of immigrants, the Amish came to the New World in search of religious freedom. Since 1900, the Old Order Amish population has grown from 5,000 to over 100,000 people (Brewer & Bonalumi, 1996).

COMMUNICATION CONSIDERATIONS

 The Amish are distinguished by their strict adherence to their traditional values and their resistance to acculturation into the white mainstream culture that surrounds them.

The Amish, who choose to live in rural farming areas, have developed settlements in over 20 states. However, approximately 75% of their total population reside in Pennsylvania, Ohio, and Indiana. Amish settlements are divided into church districts that are composed of 30 to 40 families. As church districts are only about 3 miles apart, it is easy for Amish families to travel between districts by horse and buggy, their traditional mode of transportation.

Love of family is at the center of the Amish person's life. Ideally, the three generational Amish family is composed of the father, mother, seven children, and the grandparents who help to provide child care. Although the man is the head of the family, women are respected in their roles of wife and mother. While marriages between first cousins are discouraged, the Amish tend to marry among themselves, which has lead to genetic disorders (Wenger, 1991).

As a group, the Amish strive in every way to insulate themselves and their children from worldly influences. Access to print and electronic media is restricted. Although the Amish may publish their own newsletters, they avoid exposure to secular newspapers, radio and TV programs, and the Internet. Children are educated only through the 8th grade, and then they are expected to engage in productive work on the farm. Although English is used in Amish schools, the Amish prefer to use **Deitsch** or Pennsylvania German when at home and in the community.

The Amish also dress in a manner that clearly sets them apart from other people. Homemade clothing is characterized by its plain old fashioned designs and somber colors. Women do not wear jewelry or cosmetics; they wear their long hair braided or pinned under white organdy caps, which are topped with black bonnets for outdoor wear.

Important Amish traditional values include the following (Wenger & Wenger, 1998):

- **Demut** which is German for humility. This value is expressed in the plain dress and modest demeanor of the Amish in public.

- **Gelassenheit**, German for passiveness, quiet acceptance of life, and contentment.

- Caring for the needs of others, especially for those who are ill or elderly is paramount. Helping others is *The Amish Way*.

- Conformity to the will of the group is far more important than individual rights. The Amish are cooperative, not competitive, with each other.

Filipino Values

Filipinos are the fastest growing Asian group in North America, with a United States population of 1,450,000 and a Canadian population of 157,250 people (Miranda, McBride, & Spangler, 1998). Most of the Filipinos in the United States have immigrated from the Philippine Islands, which are located in the Pacific Ocean, approximately 450 miles from the coast of China.

Over the centuries, the culture of the Philippines has been influenced by the Malaysian, Chinese, Japanese, Indonesian, and Asian Indian cultures. Philippine culture was also shaped by the Arabs who brought Islam to the

Islands in the late 1300s, and later by the Spaniards who converted the majority of Filipinos to Catholicism. In addition, American servicemen who were stationed in the Philippines during World War II brought American ideas and values to the Filipino people (Miranda, McBride, & Spangler, 1998).

Tagalog is the primary language spoken in the Philippines. The two other official languages are English and Spanish. However, within the Philippines there are approximately 75 ethnolinguistic groups who speak more than 100 languages. For the sake of simplicity, the Philippine government has given all of these languages the collective name of **Pilipino**.

The Filipino family is basically monogamous, although some **Muslim** Filipinos believe in polygamy. Husbands are titular heads of the household, but mothers have an equal say in decisions regarding family finances and the children. Because education paves the road to better jobs and higher salaries, Filipino families vigorously promote higher education for their children. Fathers and mothers willingly sacrifice to send their older children to school. The older children are then expected to help younger siblings obtain a sound education. Filipino Americans also want their children to learn Western ways in order to successfully blend in with the dominant white culture in America.

Traditional Filipino values include the following (Miranda, McBride, & Spangler, 1998):

- **Galang** or respect is the primary Filipino value. In particular, Filipinos must honor and respect their parents and elders. For example, it is important to avoid openly disagreeing with a parent or older sibling. A Filipino health care professional who immigrates to the United States may find it difficult to disagree with an administrator or physician (see Chapter 14). A person who is not respectful loses face and suffers *hiya* or shame.

- **Amor propio** is having personal pride, saving face, and avoiding hiya. One way by which Filipinos save face is to avoid arguing with older people and individuals in authority.

- Acceptance of pain and suffering is considered honorable. Some Filipinos believe that pain provides an opportunity for spiritual growth.

Iranian Values

Approximately 1 million Iranians currently live in the United States. Around 450,000 Iranians live in California; 39,000 reside in Canada. Los Angeles contains the largest population of Iranians in the world outside of Iran (Lipson & Hafizi, 1998).

Since 1980, an estimated 800,000 Iranians have migrated to the United States from Iran, formerly known as Persia. Most of these Iranian immigrants were fleeing the aftermath of the 1979 Islamic revolution and the 1980s war between Iran and Iraq (Pliskin, 1992).

Unfortunately, because of anti-American events in Iran, Iranian refugees have been subjected to ethnic bias and discrimination in the United States. Anti-Iranian sentiments ran particularly high in this country as a result of the Hostage Crisis, during which a United States Embassy in Tehran was occupied between November 1979 and January 1981 by followers of the Ayatollah Khomeini. Being forced to flee from a revolution at home to a new country where they were disliked and distrusted has adversely affected many Iranians, both physically and emotionally.

Despite these problems, Iranian immigrants (many from upper and middle class backgrounds) have been able to create a middle-class lifestyle for themselves in the United States. In the ethnic community in Los Angeles, many Iranians who were formerly physicians, engineers, or professors in Iran have gone into business for themselves. In 1987, 61% of Iranians in Los Angeles were self-employed. Many opened their own pizza parlors or gas stations, or owned their own taxicabs. Iranian women developed home-based businesses, working as seamstresses, pastry makers, beauticians, or make-up artists. Iranians have tended to avoid menial labor, as this type of work is not respected in Iran (Lipson & Hafizi, 1998).

Although the majority of Iranians who have come to the United States are Muslims, small groups of Iranians embrace Judaism, Christianity, Baha'is, and Zorasterism. Strict Muslims observe Friday as a holy day, and they strive to practice the five tenets of the Islamic faith:

1. believe in Allah

2. pray 5 times a day at designated times

3. give to the poor

4. fast during the month of Ramadan

5. make a once-in-a-lifetime pilgrimage to the holy city of Mecca in Saudi Arabia.

Many Iranian-Americans do not observe all of the traditional practices of Islam.

The Iranian family is patriarchal and hierarchical. The father is the head of the household, and he expects his wife and children to obey him. In the father's absence, the oldest son is in control. Although the status of Iranian women has improved since the 1960s' social reforms in Iran, wives are still expected to defer to their husbands and care for the home and children, even though they may be working outside the home.

Traditional Iranian values include the following:

- *Respect for higher education and advanced degrees.* Iranians are among the most highly educated immigrants in the United States.

- **Zerangi** *or cleverness.* Iranians respect the person who is able to barter and bargain in the marketplace, and consequently get the highest price possible.

- *Respect for elders.* Iranians feel that they are obligated to take care of their elderly relatives.

- *Respect for Persia's religious and artistic heritage.* Persia has produced some of the world's greatest art and poetry. Persia has also contributed to the disciplines of philosophy and medicine.

- *Modesty, respectability, and politeness.* Iranians believe that it is important to please others, be hospitable, and maintain a good reputation.

Irish Values

Irish traditions and values are a major part of American culture. Millions of Irish have immigrated to the United States over the last four centuries. Today, it is estimated that one in every five people in the United States is of Irish descent. In other words, 38.7 million people or 15.6% of the population can proudly claim an Irish heritage (Wilson, 1998).

The majority of Irish-Americans immigrated to the United States from Ireland (EIRE) between the 1600s and 1965. The Irish left their homeland to escape religious persecution, extreme poverty, and the constant threat of famine. The first settlers made their home in the Northeastern part of this country. For this reason, Boston, Philadelphia, and New York contain the largest Irish settlements in the United States. During the 1920s, 90% of the Irish lived in the cities, and they became known as the **Shanty Irish**. Later, many of the second and third generational Irish moved to the suburbs, where they became known as the **Lace Curtain Irish**.

Although the Irish suffered greatly in their homeland, life in the New World was also difficult for the new immigrants. The early Irish settlers were persecuted for their Roman Catholic faith. The majority lived hard lives in poverty. However, a strong religious faith, work ethic, and sense of humor helped the Irish survive the harsh early years in this country, and successfully assimilate into the mainstream white culture.

The traditional Irish family is patrilineal, although modern Irish families are more democratic, with all members willing to share household and child-rearing tasks. Due to their strong sense of tradition, the Irish tend to be oriented toward the past. Also, the Irish are traditionally fatalistic. Many Irish believe that humans are subject to the laws of nature and of God, and thus there is little a person can do to correct a problem. This belief may explain why some Irish tend to deny and ignore illnesses and pain.

Traditional Irish values include the following:

- *Obligation and devotion to the family.* Traditionally, the Irish have valued large families with many children.

- *Strong faith in God.* The majority of Irish-Americans are Roman Catholics.

- *Respect for the elderly.* The Irish value the advice and experience of the elderly.

- *Education and hard work.* The Irish are well represented in law, medicine, science, and literature. The Irish have also risen to prominence in politics.

- *Accepting life's difficulties with humor.* The Irish are known for their humor, wit, and ability to write biting social satire.

Jewish Values

The word *Jew* is defined in *Webster's Dictionary* as "(1) one who is descended or regarded as descended from the ancient Hebrews, and (2) one whose religion is Judaism." The practice of Judaism ranges from liberal Reform to Orthodox. **Orthodox Jews** recognize the child who is born to a Jewish mother as a Jew. **Reform Jews** are more liberal, and they also recognize the child who is born to a Jewish father and a non-Jewish mother as Jewish (Selekman, 1998).

Jewish people do not belong to a race, nor do they belong to any one nationality. People who call themselves Jews come from all over the world. **Ashkenazi** (Yiddish for German) **Jews** come from Eastern Europe and Russia; 82% of Jews are of Ashkenazi descent. **Sephardic Jews** come from Spain, Portugal, the Mediterranean area, Africa, Central America, and South America. **Sabras** are Jews born in Israel.

Although the Jewish people have highly diverse backgrounds, Jews also have a great deal in common. Jews share religious beliefs, cultural values, family traditions, and common folk traditions. Jews also share a long and painful history of persecution. The Jewish people have suffered tremendous losses of life, liberty, and property during, for example, the anti-Jewish riots (**pogroms**) in Russia and Eastern Europe, and the **Holocaust** in Nazi Germany and Poland. Even those Jews who immigrated to the United States in search of freedom and peace faced prejudice and anti-Semitism in their new homeland.

Currently, approximately 5.7 million Jews (around 1% of the world Jewish population) live in the United States (Selekman, 1998). The Jewish immigrants primarily settled in the Northeast. Today, Jews live in large cities all over this country; for example, Los Angeles, New York, Miami, and Boston. As a group, Jewish Americans have attained professional respect and economic success. As the Jews greatly value higher education and advanced degrees, many Jewish-Americans are professional people who excel as lawyers, physicians, dentists, scientists, and university professors.

In addition to education and work, Jewish life revolves around religion and family life. Judaism is a **monotheistic** faith (belief in one God) primarily based on the **Torah**, or first five books of the Bible, also known as the Books of Moses. The rabbi is the spiritual leader of the Jews. Jewish services are held in a synagogue, temple, or shul, where prayer is conducted in Hebrew. In America, Judaism is divided into 3 major denominations:

1. Orthodox Jews adhere strictly to the traditions of Judaism, the traditional Code of Jewish Law, and dietary laws that state which foods are **kosher** (fit for eating) and which foods are **treyf** (forbidden or unclean). **Hasidic Jews** are ultra-Orthodox traditionalists who rigidly follow strict rules in their dress, living arrangements, and religious practices.

2. **Conservative Jews** follow many of the Orthodox Jewish traditions, but are less strict in their adherence to Jewish mores.

3. Reform Jews are much more liberal in their beliefs and practices than Orthodox and Conservative Jews. For example, Reform Jews may not observe traditional dietary practices.

Jewish family life depends upon which branch of Judaism is practiced by family members. Traditional or Orthodox Jewish families are definitely male-oriented, whereas the families of Conservative and Reform Jews are more equalitarian. Jewish marriages are monogamous. Jewish parents welcome children as blessings, and they strive to provide their offspring with love, a religious upbringing, and an excellent education.

Traditional Jewish values include the following:

- Higher education and continued learning throughout life

- **Tzedakah** or righteousness and sharing. Jewish people value being charitable and generous towards those who are in need

- *Respect for parents and elders.* Jews believe that it is important to honor their fathers and mothers and to care for their elderly parents and relatives

- *Modesty and humility.* These virtues are particularly valued by Orthodox Jews

- *Humor.* As a way to cope with bias and prejudice, Jews value the ability to laugh at a situation and at themselves

- *Good health.* When ill, Jews value regaining their health to such a degree that they may waive traditional practices (such as dietary laws), if these practices might interfere with the healing process

TESTING YOUR KNOWLEDGE

Circle the correct answer.

1. An orientation toward the future is particularly valued by
   a. Asian culture.
   b. white mainstream American culture.
   c. Hispanic culture.
   d. Native American culture.

2. Shintoism is primarily practiced by the
   a. Chinese.
   b. Japanese.
   c. Koreans.
   d. Vietnamese.

3. Native Americans particularly value
   a. orientation to the present.
   b. extended family.
   c. cooperation.
   d. all of the above.

4. Humility is an important virtue for which of the following cultures?
   a. Jewish
   b. Amish
   c. Irish
   d. black

5. Tagalog is a primary language of
   a. Japan.
   b. Indochina.
   c. the Philippines.
   d. Samoa.

6. Zerangi (cleverness) is highly respected by
   a. Jewish culture
   b. white mainstream culture.
   c. Iranian culture.
   d. black culture.

7. Hasidic Jews are classified as
   a. Orthodox.
   b. Conservative.
   c. Reform.
   d. Ultra-orthodox traditionalists.

3

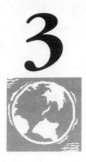

TRANSCULTURAL COMMUNICATION BUILDING BLOCKS: BELIEFS, BEHAVIOR, AND COMMUNICATION

KEY TERMS

- Acceptable Behavior
- Alternative Health Care System
- Biomedical Belief System
- Biomedical Health Care System
- Communication
- Folk Sector
- Holistic Belief System
- Language
- Medical Pluralism
- Mind–Body Dichotomy
- Nonverbal Communication
- Popular Health Care System
- Proxemics
- Supernatural Belief System
- Verbal Communication

OBJECTIVES

After completing this chapter, you should be able to:

- Specify the ways in which major *health belief systems* differ.
- Specify the ways in which major *health care systems* differ.
- Discuss how cultural similarities affect behavior.
- Discuss cultural diversity; in other words, describe factors other than culture that dictate how each individual within a culture behaves.

- Recognize that different cultures use different verbal communication styles.

- Recognize that different cultures use various forms of nonverbal communication.

- More accurately assess clients' verbal and nonverbal responses to pain, fear, and illness.

INTRODUCTION

Recall from Chapter 2 that transcultural communication is built, first of all, on culture. Culture, in turn, forms the basis for values. *Cultural values* (which we explore in this chapter), support the beliefs and behaviors that are accepted within each culture. Beliefs and behaviors, in turn, influence communication patterns—both verbal and nonverbal—within different cultures.

Health care professionals come into contact with people from many diverse cultures and walks of life. To provide culturally competent care, health care professionals must recognize and accept clients with different belief systems and styles of behavior. Moreover, health care professionals must be able to speak with clients who have different communication styles, and who may have limited proficiency in English.

BELIEFS

Like value systems, belief systems are heavily influenced by culture. Beliefs, in turn, guide human behavior and communication. Important belief systems include religious, ethical, and political beliefs. For health care professionals, the cultural belief systems that govern health, illness, and health care are of greatest importance.

Different cultures have different beliefs about what causes illness, what should be done to identify illness, and how to treat illness. For instance, is a disease caused by a microorganism, or an evil spirit, or a disharmony in nature? Is disease most accurately diagnosed by physical assessment, laboratory studies, or by the interpretation of dreams?

Cultural beliefs also influence how individuals within a culture define health and disease. For example, a truck driver in Los Angeles might regard a worm infestation as a sign of illness, but ignore symptoms from the smog. On the other hand, a man from the island of Tristan da Cunha might acknowledge that the smog in Los Angeles makes him ill, but ignore a worm infestation because it is so common on his island.

Beliefs also guide the choices people make when they seek symptom relief and the cure for illness. Will the person seek out a medical doctor (MD) or instead go to the pharmacy and purchase over-the-counter drugs? Or will the individual turn to a religious leader or a practitioner of alternative medicine? How each of us deals with disease depends upon what we believe causes disease, and who we believe is most qualified to treat disease.

Health Belief Systems

The three major types of health belief systems are

1. biomedical
2. supernatural
3. holistic

The **biomedical belief system** arose from the teachings of René Descartes, a 17th century philosopher. Descartes conceived of each person as a body machine. This mechanistic theory produced the concept of dualism or the **mind–body dichotomy**; that is, the mind and body are separate from each other. According to this model, disease is caused by physiologic disturbances such as genetic disorders, biochemical imbalances, and infectious organisms. Pathologic alterations in tissues constitute evidence of disease.

As a result of their biomedical training, biomedical practitioners pay primary attention to physical complaints and pathophysiologic changes. At the same time, these practitioners de-emphasize mental and emotional problems and the psychosocial component of disease. Traditional treatment usually involves administering medications or performing surgery.

Western physicians have introduced biomedicine into numerous cultures around the world. This belief system continues to dominate diagnostics and health care throughout the United States.

The **supernatural belief system**, widely accepted in traditional Hispanic, Caribbean, African, and other cultures, differs dramatically from the biomedical model. Cultural groups that believe in the supernatural model may view illness as a sign of weakness, a punishment for evil-doing, or retribution for shameful behavior such as disrespect toward elders. Some cultures also believe that illness results from the possession of the body by evil spirits or from the casting of evil spells.

Example: A 10-year-old boy from a rural Mexican family was being treated for an osteosarcoma of his distal femur. He had been transported to a medical center from a village health clinic. According to the father, his son's cancer began when the boy was kicked by a child from a neighboring family with whom the father was feuding.

The father believed that his neighbors had cast an evil spell, causing a snake to invade his son, and thus the child had developed an illness as a result of the kick. Because the father believed there was a supernatural cause for his son's illness, he also believed that the evil spell would have to be removed for the boy to be cured.

To diagnose illness, some Hispanics who have traditional values might consult with a *curandero* (healer); people in Caribbean cultures might go to a Voodoo priest or priestess. Other cultures (for example, some Native Americans) traditionally rely on dreams and divination. Traditional Native American health care professionals sometimes enter a trance state to understand a person's symptoms.

In a phenomenon called **medical pluralism** or dual use, some Native Americans turn to a medicine man to determine the true cause of an illness (i.e., why the person is out of harmony with nature) as well as to a Western physician to determine the immediate cause of the illness. Dual use or medical pluralism is not limited to any specific cultural group. Many individuals seek and use more than one system of care.

Example: A young Alaskan native woman who lived in a large city and regularly saw a health care professional would also return to her village for teas and herbs. She sought these remedies for a lingering condition that had not improved with biomedical treatment.

To treat illness, traditional healers who believe in the supernatural may rely on sorcery, prayer, magic, and witchcraft—using religious rites, amulets, masks, and sand painting. They may beseech their deceased ancestors or the spirit world to heal the ill person. This type of belief system also appears in the mainstream culture, despite a strong reliance on the biomedical belief system. Western Christians and Jews often turn to God when faced with life threatening illnesses that biomedical doctors cannot cure.

The **holistic belief system** is primarily upheld by Asian cultures and some Native American cultures, although holistic beliefs have started to infiltrate traditional Western thinking. Disenchanted with the biomedical emphasis on technology, medications, and curing illness, a growing number of Americans are now interested in the concept of holistic medicine with its emphasis on health promotion.

Unlike Western medicine, the holistic system emphasizes illness prevention and health maintenance. The major premise of this system is that there are natural laws that govern everything and every person in the universe. To be healthy, a person must remain in harmony with the natural laws and be willing to continually adjust and adapt to changes in the environment.

According to this system, illness develops when one does not properly care for the body; for example, we subject ourselves to too much cold, too much heat, too much alcohol, or an improper diet. In essence, illness results when a person fails to act in harmony with nature, causing vital elements within the body to become imbalanced. The Chinese culture refers to these elements as *yin* and *yang,* while the Hispanic and Eastern Mediterranean cultural groups use the terms *hot* and *cold.* Too much of either of these elements (yin, yang, heat, cold) causes illness.

To restore health, the person must restore equilibrium to the body. Thus, in some cultures, people may use hot remedies if they have too much cold, or cold remedies if too much heat. For instance, if a client's headache is thought to be caused by a hot agent, (fever, infection, diarrhea, constipation) then the person is treated with cold foods such as fresh vegetables, tropical fruits, barley, water, and cold medicines such as milk of magnesia or bicarbonate of soda.

Health Care Systems

There are four health care systems that are related to the health belief systems just described:

1. the biomedical health care system
2. the popular health care system
3. the folk or traditional health care system
4. the alternative health care system

Within the United States, many people use all of the systems, either individually, in combination, or simultaneously.

The **biomedical health care system** combines the Western biomedical beliefs that originated with Descartes and the traditional American values of self-reliance, individualism, and aggressive action. This system is geared to conquer disease by battling the onslaught of microorganisms and diseased cells, as well as the breakdown of the body's organs due to aging. The American values of aggression, mastery over one's own fate, and dominance over nature are expressed in such phrases as "conquering disease," "winning the battle against cancer," or "beating AIDS."

The American medical system is composed of health care professionals who have received specialized biomedical training and are legally and officially recognized as professionals. Licensed care providers may diagnose clients, legally prescribe and administer medications, and perform surgery. In recent years, biomedical care providers have shifted from a narrow focus on treating diseases to the broader avenues of disease prevention and health promotion.

Consistent with Western values of self-reliance and individualism, the American medical system encourages clients to learn as much as possible about their illnesses. This open information policy extends to the prognosis for a critical illness. Even when a disease may be terminal, many American physicians feel that clients have a right to know the facts about their condition, and what treatment options, if any, are open to them.

Conversely, Japanese physicians are hesitant to tell clients that they have a terminal disease, preferring to keep silent, and thus sustain hope. Physicians in Bangladesh might merely suggest that terminal clients eat whatever they choose. In this way, the physician can subtly convey that the client will probably not recover.

Teaching clients self-care is also an important component of Western medicine. For example, Western health care professionals routinely teach clients to give themselves insulin injections, change their own dressings, and self-administer medications. In contrast, health care professionals from Taiwan, where a collective orientation is more common, expect family members to actively care for the client.

The **popular health care system**, which involves self-treatment, is the first source of care most people use, regardless of culture. For instance, the average person who has cold or flu symptoms (or has a child with such symptoms) does not initially call a physician. Instead the sick individual goes to the drug store and buys a cold or flu remedy. If the remedy fails and symptoms worsen, the person may next call friends and relatives for advice on home or drug store remedies. Only when all else fails will the person consider calling the doctor or going to a clinic.

Popular health care is also the basis for self-care groups such as Alcoholics Anonymous and various cancer support groups. Although it is often overlooked by biomedical health care professionals, popular health care provides a major source of care for a variety of problems and complaints.

The **folk sector** or *traditional medicine sector* includes various folk healers who use a variety of treatment modalities. Folk healers include shamans, herbalists, acupressurists, and acupuncturists. Folk healers usually maintain a holistic approach and endeavor to treat the whole person within the context of the family. Care planning and treatment take into consideration the social, physiologic, and spiritual dimensions of the client. Folk healers are trained in their roles, and they usually have a high status in their cultural group.

Clients and their families may often move between popular, folk, and biomedical systems in various patterns of help-seeking behavior. Clients might initially select popular remedies, and then shift to alternative sources of care. They may ultimately seek a biomedical practitioner only if other approaches fail. Conversely, clients may initially seek biomedical care, but might then resort to folk modalities and popular treatments in light of a perceived lack of success.

Another system is the **alternative health care system**. Although they vary greatly, alternative medical practices have two common traits: (1) they differ from biomedical beliefs, and (2) they evaluate success differently from biomedical research methods.

Practitioners of alternative medicine include chiropractors, homeopaths, naturopaths, and hypnotists. Examples of alternative health care are:

1. *Diet therapy:* macrobiotics and megavitamins

2. *Mind/body control methods:* relaxation, counseling, prayer, hypnotherapy, and guided imagery

3. *Methods working with body structure and energy:* chiropractic, massage, and therapeutic touch

4. *Pharmacologic and biologic therapies:* antioxidants, oxidizing agents, and chelation therapy

Many Americans are choosing to try alternative medicine. According to a national survey published in *The Landmark Report on Public Perceptions of Alternative Care* (1998), 42% of the 1500 adults interviewed had used some form of alternative care during 1996 and 1997. Of these individuals

• 74% had used alternative care *in addition* to traditional care.

• 15% had *replaced* traditional care with alternative care.

• 11% had used alternative care along with *and* as a replacement for traditional care.

Respondents were also asked how important the *availability* of alternative care was for them when choosing a health plan. Of the respondents

• 31% felt that alternative care was *very important* when choosing a health plan.

• 36% felt that alternative care was *somewhat important* when choosing a health plan.

• 33% felt that alternative care was *not important* when choosing a health plan.

Finally, researchers attempted to forecast the outlook for alternative care by asking respondents if they had experienced any *change of opinion* toward alternative care over the past five years. Of the respondents

• 40% stated that their opinion toward alternative care had grown *more positive.*

• 58% stated that their opinion of alternative care had *not changed.*

• 2% stated that their opinion of alternative care had become *more negative.*

BEHAVIOR

Cultural values dictate human behavior to a vast extent. Culture encourages each of us to think, feel, and then act in certain prescribed ways—thus the reason for cultural similarities. On the other hand, each culture is made up of individuals whose beliefs and behavior reflect some aspects of their culture, but not all aspects—thus the reason for cultural diversity.

Cultural Similarities

Culture encourages us to behave in a way similar to others in our culture while behaving quite differently from people of other cultures. Indeed, people are consciously or subconsciously rewarded for being with and acting like people who resemble themselves.

Example: Most middle-class Americans are culturally conditioned to eat three meals a day, work 5 days a week, and celebrate certain holidays at specific times of the year according to definite traditions (Christmas, Easter, 4th of July, Thanksgiving). But those from other cultures—especially Asia and Africa—have vastly different eating, working, and celebrating habits, and they may view traditional Western activities with skepticism.

Culture dictates what is **acceptable behavior** when sick. Identifying what is acceptable behavior within your client's culture will help you understand your client's reactions to illness. In some cultures (e.g., Asian and Native American cultures), clients are expected to be stoic and silent when in pain. On the other hand, within the Mediterranean culture, it is acceptable to express pain with loud complaints and dramatic gestures.

Culture also influences whether or not a person is willing to talk about their symptoms or emotions with health care professionals. For instance, Asian cultures typically value a subtle approach to problems and the restraint of strong feelings. Thus Asian clients may find it difficult to speak openly about symptoms or emotional problems with strangers. Conversely, middle class white Americans, raised in a society that values open expression, may welcome an opportunity to frankly discuss their symptoms with health care professionals.

Like larger cultures, subcultures also foster similar behavior patterns among members. These behavior patterns are based on specific subcultural values and beliefs. The health care profession has its own organizations and educational programs that clarify goals and behaviors, creating a health care subculture.

Clients seeking health care also form a subculture. Clients are expected to conform to hospital, office, or institutional policies, and conform to the schedule of the health care facility. Furthermore, clients are asked to cheerfully endure invasions of their privacy for the sake of their health. People who enter a health care facility for treatment must put aside their usual roles (mother, businessman, teacher) and behave as a client within the health care subculture.

Cultural Diversity

Although each culture dictates general values and behavior among its members, factors other than culture dictate how each individual within that culture should behave. Important factors that influence behavior patterns and habits include:

1. Age
2. Gender
3. Length of residence in the United States
4. Rural or urban residence
5. Occupation
6. Level of education
7. Use of English
8. Degree of acculturation
9. Socioeconomic class
10. Personality characteristics
11. Previous experiences
12. Personal beliefs
13. Religious beliefs

Example: Suppose you were asked to predict what a typical middle-class white American would have for dinner. Your chances of predicting the meal accurately would be better if you knew the person's age (is the person a teenager who loves junk food?), socioeconomic status (is steak too expensive?), religion (is pork permitted?), personal experiences (does the person identify a home-cooked chicken dinner with a happy home life?) and personal beliefs (is the person a vegetarian?). So many individual factors other than culture play a role in selecting a meal that it is impossible to know the menu for a typical American dinner.

Likewise, when caring for clients from different cultures, remember that culture only provides the broad canvas of information upon which each person paints the details of his or her personality and life experiences. Even if you are an expert on a client's culture, you will not be able to predict exactly how that person is going to behave when ill. The person's educational level, presence or lack of support systems, degree of medical knowledge, past experiences with illness and hospitalization, and many other factors will ultimately determine how that individual will respond to illness.

COMMUNICATION CONSIDERATIONS

Remember to recognize the individuality of each client, regardless of culture.

COMMUNICATION

At its most basic level, **communication** occurs when a person (the sender or encoder) sends a message to another person (the receiver or decoder). The message may be **verbal** (spoken or written in a language), or **nonverbal** (conveyed through facial expressions and/or body language). Communication is most effective when the message received is exactly the same as the message that was sent and both sender and receiver agree on the meaning of the message.

Communication fails when (1) the sender's message is blocked for some reason and the receiver never gets the message, or (2) the message is distorted. Distortion occurs when the message has a different meaning for the receiver than the sender intended. Distortion is amplified when the sender and receiver fail to seek feedback and clarify the message. Factors that can distort messages include anger, fatigue, fear, pain, and anxiety.

Moreover, communication may be blocked when senders and receivers come from different cultural, ethnic, racial, socioeconomic, or educational backgrounds. For example, Japanese Americans with a traditional background may not want to question or challenge health care professionals especially physicians. As a result, some Japanese American clients may silently accept a physician's recommendations even when they do not understand the reasons for the medications or procedures that are ordered.

Verbal Communication

Verbal communication, which includes both the spoken and written word, depends upon language. **Language** is the code senders use to carry their messages.

COMMUNICATION CONSIDERATIONS

Language allows us to initially identify, label, attach significance to, and evaluate our experiences.

Language barriers can create severe communication problems between senders and receivers. Language barriers may arise from the use of different language systems (e.g., the sender is speaking English and the receiver is speaking Spanish), or they can arise when the sender uses technical terms, abbreviations, idioms, or regionalisms that are unfamiliar to the receiver (e.g., when a health care professional uses medical terms when explaining a procedure to a lay person).

Every culture has *standards* for verbal communication—especially for word choice, inflection, volume and speed of speech, directness, and the degree of emotion considered appropriate.

Word Choice. American speech is filled with abbreviated words, slang, and jargon. Americans tend to communicate in an informal way with superiors and subordinates alike. In contrast, the Japanese use of language is distinguished by many levels of formality and degrees of politeness, depending upon the status of the people who are conversing. The Japanese also make distinctions between men's and women's speech. Thus the choice of words for the Japanese depends largely on the relationship between the people who are communicating. An expression such as "What is this?" can be said in several different ways, depending on the sender's relationship to the receiver.

Emotional Expressiveness, Tone, Pitch, Volume of Voice, and Speed of Speech. Traditionally, black and white American cultures differ in the amount of expressiveness allowed when verbally communicating. For example, white American middle-class culture values a controlled tone of voice and some emotional restraint. On the other hand, many black Americans are more verbal and value emotional expressiveness in a conversation or discussion. Because of this difference in values, middle-class whites may not understand that blacks tend to express themselves dynamically, and thus misinterpret their loud voice volume as aggression (Campinha-Bacote, 1998).

However, even whites vary in the emotion and expression in their voices. For instance, Appalachians characteristically speak very slowly, and they seem to dwell on each word, giving their speech a hesitant, disjointed quality. Unlike blacks and whites, many Asians and Native Americans display great emotional restraint in their speech patterns, speaking slowly and quietly. These cultures may value the ability to endure pain and grief with silent stoicism.

In marked contrast, Southern Europeans are typically warm, expressive, and sometimes dramatic in both their verbal and nonverbal communication. Generally they are not stoic about pain, but will loudly express their discomfort. People from more expressive cultures may view Asians and Native Americans as withdrawn, shy, and silent.

Voice Inflection. When one person talks to another, the emphasis that is placed on certain words often says more than the words themselves. For example, "What do you *need* now?" sends a different message from "What do you need *now?*" In many languages, the inflection given to the syllables of some words can change the meaning.

Directness In Speech. When communicating, some cultures value politeness more than others. Americans, being members of an impatient and future-oriented culture, like to get to the point of a conversation rather than wasting time on lengthy preliminaries or long silences. Americans may be quite direct when communicating with others. Mexicans, on the other hand, strive to be polite, diplomatic, and tactful. They may take the time for small talk, and then lead into a discussion.

Use Of Silence. Some cultures value silence whereas other cultural groups feel that silence is a vacuum that must immediately be filled with words. Among some Native Americans, silence is an essential element of showing respect and understanding. In some Arab cultures, silence may indicate concern for personal privacy. The French, Spanish, and Soviet cultures interpret silence as a sign of agreement. Silence during a conversation also gives each person an opportunity to speak without having to interrupt.

Nonverbal Communication

Experts estimate that as much as two-thirds of all communication is nonverbal, consisting of messages that are conveyed from one person to another via body language and facial expressions. Specific forms of nonverbal communication throughout the world include the examples that follow.

Gestures and Facial Expressions. The world's many cultures differ vastly in their interpretation of some gestures and facial expressions, whereas the interpretation of other gestures is fairly standard. For example, in nearly all cultures, people use their mouths and eyebrows to convey surprise, anger, pleasure, and fear, while they use hand gestures to convey openness or intimidation. Common types of nonverbal communication may differ in meaning from culture to culture. The same words that may be "read" as an insult if the speaker is glaring, might be understood to be teasing if the speaker is smiling.

Eye Movement and Eye Contact. There is an old saying that "The eyes are the windows of the soul." Because the eyes are thought to reveal a person's true nature, many Americans assume that it is a negative sign when a person avoids eye contact. It is not unusual to hear an American say "Look at me when I talk to you" or "She must be lying. Did you notice that she avoided looking at us?" American health care professionals usually note if a client avoids eye contact when they perform a psychosocial assessment.

Other cultures view the significance of eye contact differently. Some Asians and Native Americans believe that prolonged eye contact is rude and an invasion of privacy. Native Americans may divert their eyes to the floor when they are paying attention or thinking. Muslim women may avoid eye contact as a show of modesty. Appalachians tend to avoid eye contact because they feel that it expresses hostility and aggressiveness. In India, the amount of eye contact that is appropriate depends on one's social position (people of different socioeconomic classes avoid eye contact with each other).

COMMUNICATION CONSIDERATION

In Western cultures, prolonged eye contact may be considered a sign of intimacy, especially in conjunction with the use of touch. Health care professionals need to guard against prolonged eye contact with clients when performing invasive procedures.

Use of Personal and Interpersonal Space (Proxemics). The amount of personal space that people need as a comfort zone varies from individual to individual and from culture to culture. For Western culture, research has identified the following 4 zones of interpersonal space (Geiger & Davidhizar, 1995):

1. *Intimate space:* from contact to 18 inches. This space is normally reserved for people who are in close relationships. Health care professionals frequently occupy this space as they bathe and feed clients.

2. *Personal space:* from 18 inches to 4 feet. This space is commonly used for interaction between friends. It is also useful for client counseling.
3. *Social space:* from 4 to 12 feet. The business of everyday life is most often conducted within social space.
4. *Public space:* greater than 12 feet. This space is used during lectures and speeches.

Typically, middle-class Americans, Canadians, and the British feel uncomfortable when forced into close proximity with people they do not know well. In fact, white Americans who feel that their personal space is being violated may react with anger and withdrawal. Other cultures welcome physical closeness. Latin Americans, Africans, black Americans, Indonesians, Arabs, and the French prefer to stand close to one another when holding a conversation.

Problems can arise when, for example, a North American from a British background speaks with a Latin American. The North American, feeling that his personal space is being violated, may find himself backing away from his Latin American acquaintance. The Latin American may interpret the North American's reaction as a sign of aloofness, dislike, or unwillingness to talk. In reality, the problem is not one of personalities, but of proxemics.

Touch. Depending on whether it is gentle, sensual, harsh, or brutal, touch conveys many meanings. We use touch to connect with others and establish feelings of warmth, approval, emotional support, and intimacy. On the other hand, touch can communicate anger, aggression, frustration, and a desire to control others by invading their personal space. Touch (or a laying on of hands) may also be regarded as therapeutic.

Cultures have specific guidelines for times and situations when it is acceptable to touch others. Middle-class Americans typically consummate a business deal with a handshake; some Native Americans, however, view a firm handshake as aggressive and even offensive. Many Westerners think nothing of kissing or hugging a friend as a form of greeting when meeting in public places. In traditional Asian cultures, such behavior is reserved for intimate relationships.

Posture. Posture helps to communicate how one person feels toward another. For instance, middle-class Americans may lean in the direction of individuals that they like or respect. Posture can also communicate a tense or relaxed state. Crossed arms tend to distance the parties in an interaction, whereas greeting someone with open arms suggests a desire to be close to that person. Rigid muscles and a flexed body may indicate physical pain.

COMMUNICATION CONSIDERATIONS

Be aware of the client's verbal and nonverbal communications as well as inconsistencies between them.

The message conveyed by nonverbal communication may be far closer to the truth than verbal communication. For example, the man who pounds on the table and shouts "I'm not angry!" is clearly showing his anger. The pre-operative client who looks worried and tense but tells you she is not afraid of surgery is showing her fear through her expressions and body language.

You also need to observe for communication that is *vocal but still nonverbal*. This universal type of communication includes moaning, sighing, gasping, crying, laughing, and coughing.

Assessing Verbal and Nonverbal Responses

The various communication styles that arise from cultural differences can make it difficult for health care professionals to accurately assess their clients' verbal and nonverbal responses to illness or surgery. It can be particularly challenging to evaluate clients' responses to pain.

Example: Karen Green, a young physical therapist, was involved in providing a rehabilitative program for two clients following hip replacement surgery. Mrs. Wong, a middle-aged Chinese woman who had been in the United States for five years and spoke limited English always declined Karen's offers of mild pain relievers during therapy sessions. Mrs. Wong's face looked tense and drawn and her attempts to move through therapy were very guarded.

Mrs. Tortano was a middle-aged Italian-American woman who had spent her entire life in the city's Italian community. She often clutched Karen's hand and shouted, "Give me a shot! I can't stand the pain!" Karen noted that at these times Mrs. Tortano would clutch her hip and leg and refuse to participate further in therapy.

Even though each woman expressed her discomfort differently, Karen concluded that both of her clients were experiencing severe pain that required medication. The fact that pain can evoke such different verbal and nonverbal responses may be due to personality or cultural differences or both.

Karen had learned that Asian cultures value a more stoic response to pain, while the Italian culture tolerates a more emotive response to pain. Karen also recognized that individuals do not necessarily conform to the communication style accepted in their culture. Thus some Asians may be more emotive, and some Italians more stoic when dealing with pain, grief, and other difficult circumstances.

COMMUNICATION CONSIDERATIONS

Clients from different cultures may communicate their pain, anxiety, fear, and other powerful feelings and emotions in different ways. Thus health care professionals need to carefully assess their clients in order to accurately decode their transcultural communication—both verbal and nonverbal.

Techniques for eliciting assessment data from clients from different cultures is discussed in detail in Chapter 10.

TESTING YOUR KNOWLEDGE

Circle the correct answer.

1. The holistic health belief system
   a. is primarily upheld by Hispanic and black American cultures.
   b. is rarely accepted by middle-class White Americans.
   c. utilizes such elements as *yin* and *yang*.
   d. emphasizes self-care.

2. In what important way does the Western biomedical system diverge from other systems of care, including traditional Native American healing?
   a. reliance on spiritual guidance
   b. extensive questioning, and the use of examination and laboratory techniques
   c. reliance on intuitive knowledge
   d. extensive use of secondary data

3. The loudness and intensity of speech among blacks from primarily black communities, is usually an indication of
   a. anger.
   b. emotional expressiveness.
   c. confusion.
   d. resentment.

4. In the 1998 *Landmark Report on Public Perceptions of Alternative Care*, approximately how many respondents had used some type of alternative care during 1996 and 1997?
   a. 10% of respondents
   b. 20% of respondents
   c. 30% of respondents
   d. 40% of respondents

5. Direct eye contact is usually considered acceptable in which one of the following cultures?
   a. Native American
   b. White North American
   c. Appalachian
   d. Asian

6. In Western culture, there are 4 zones of interpersonal space. *Personal space* is measured from
   a. contact with another person to 18 inches.
   b. 18 inches to 4 feet.
   c. 4 feet to 6 feet.
   d. 6 feet to 12 feet.

CHAPTER 4

TRANSCULTURAL COMMUNICATION STUMBLING BLOCKS

KEY TERMS

- Barriers
- Biased
- Cultural Blind Spot Syndrome
- Dialect
- Ethnocentrism
- Idiom

- Health Care Rituals
- Racism
- Regionalism
- Simultaneous Dual Ethnocentrism
- Stereotype

OBJECTIVES

After completing this chapter, you should be able to:

- Identify barriers to effective transcultural communication between clients and health care professionals.
- Describe the process by which people from diverse cultures go from fearing each other to liking each other.
- Identify and describe the three types of racism that are found in our society.

- Define ethnocentrism and explain how this barrier blocks transcultural communication.
- Describe the different types of language barriers that can impede transcultural communication.
- Develop an awareness of the various dialects, regionalisms, and idioms that distinguish the speech of people from different races, ethnic groups, and regions.
- Identify ways in which differing perceptions and expectations can complicate communications between health care professionals and clients from diverse cultures.

INTRODUCTION

Communication between health care professionals and clients from different cultures is often complicated by different values, beliefs, traditions, expectations, and languages. As you work with clients from multicultural backgrounds, you will find that these differences raise barriers to transcultural communication. This chapter discusses communication barriers in terms of their underlying dynamics, and their impact on health care professionals, clients, and client care. Chapter 8 describes practical strategies for overcoming transcultural communication barriers in the health care arena.

BARRIERS TO TRANSCULTURAL COMMUNICATION

There are eight important **barriers** to transcultural communication in the health care setting: (1) lack of knowledge, (2) fear and distrust, (3) racism, (4) bias and ethnocentrism, (5) stereotyping, (6) ritualistic behavior, (7) language barriers, and (8) differences in perceptions and expectations.

Lack of Knowledge

The failure to understand cultural differences in values, behaviors, and communication styles is a common stumbling block for individuals who work in transcultural settings. Health care professionals who are not knowledgeable about cultural differences risk misinterpreting clients' attempts to communicate. As a result, clients may not receive the proper care.

Remember that each culture dictates what is "normal" behavior when sick; for example, Japanese clients might react with silent obedience to your requests, white middle-class clients might wish to discuss their care options with you, Italian clients might dramatically express their discomfort, while an inner city youth might loudly demand your attention. Health care professionals who are unaware of cultural differences may mistakenly expect all clients to communicate in the same way, regardless of culture.

Furthermore, health care professionals who have not learned about which behaviors are acceptable in different cultures may attribute a client's behavior (e.g., silence, withdrawal) to the wrong reason or cause—resulting in faulty assessment and intervention.

Example: A dental assistant was teaching a basic dental hygiene class to a group of white, Hispanic, and black adolescents. The dental assistant used some words that Bonita, a Hispanic teenager, did not understand. Bonita asked the dental assistant to explain what the words meant. The dental assistant, who wanted to cover the rest of her lesson, told Bonita that she would talk with her about the words after class. But when class was over, Bonita abruptly left the room.

The dental assistant, who was not knowledgeable about Hispanic culture, incorrectly assumed that Bonita had either forgotten that she was to remain after class, or had decided that she had more important things to do.

Had the dental assistant known more about the culture and behavioral patterns of Hispanics, she would have realized that:

- Hispanics typically view health care professionals and teachers as authority figures and expect them to initiate actions. Thus Bonita expected the dental assistant to call her name and remind her to stay after class.
- Many Hispanic children receive a great deal of close supervision and attention from adults. Bonita might have felt that she should not have been made to wait until after class to receive answers to her questions.
- Hispanic children are raised to be respectful and quiet. Bonita overcame her shyness when she asked the dental assistant a question. If the dental assistant had known more about the behavioral patterns of Hispanic children, she would have invited Bonita to ask her questions again at the end of class. As Bonita did not receive a cue from the dental assistant that it was all right to speak, she assumed it would be rude to raise her hand.

Thus, the dental assistant incorrectly attributed Bonita's behavior to forgetfulness or disrespect. Because the dental assistant did not understand the culturally-based reasons for Bonita's behavior, she missed a valuable opportunity to expand Bonita's grasp of dental hygiene.

Fear and Distrust

Fear, dislike, and distrust are emotions that all too often erupt when people from diverse cultures first meet. Rothenburger (1990) has identified seven stages of adjustment that individuals pass through during their initial encounters with people of different cultures that they do not know or understand. These stages are:

1. *Fear:* When first meeting someone from a different culture, many people feel threatened. Each person perceives the other person as different and, therefore, dangerous. Usually as people become better acquainted with each other, the fear gradually dissipates, only to be replaced by dislike.

2. *Dislike:* Dislike is a much milder emotion than fear. Group members have a tendency to dislike people who behave or communicate differently from what is considered "the norm" in that culture or group. For example, a working class black person might dislike a middle-class white person because white people tend to be less vocal and expressive than many black people, and thus appear insincere and weak.

3. *Distrust:* People from different cultures are often suspicious of each others' actions and motives because they lack information. For example, a white nursing assistant who does not realize the importance of family in Vietnam, may be suspicious of the new Vietnamese nursing assistant who allows family members to participate in a client's care instead of providing all of the care herself. Unfortunately, unless there is pressure to change their attitudes, some people never do progress beyond fear, dislike, and distrust to the next stage of acceptance.

4. *Acceptance:* Usually if two people from different cultures share enough good experiences over a period of time, they will begin to accept each other rather than resent each other.

5. *Respect:* If individuals from diverse cultures are open minded, they will allow themselves to see and admire qualities in one another. For example, a Japanese physical therapist who has been trained to defer to authority might admire the white American physical therapist who challenges authority. Acceptance and admiration, in turn, foster respect.

6. *Trust:* Once people from diverse cultures have spent enough quality time together, they usually are able to trust each other. For example, a white American medical assistant will eventually trust the foreign-born medical assistant who consistently provides good client care and finishes assignments on time. Once people trust each other, they may finally learn to genuinely like each other.

7. *Like:* For people to like each other, they must share many things in common. To reach this final stage, individuals from diverse cultures must be able to concentrate on the human qualities that bind people together, rather than the differences that pull people apart.

This evolution of a relationship from fear to trust has been dramatized in films. For instance *The Defiant Ones* starring Tony Curtis and Sidney Poitier is the story of two escaped convicts—one white and one black—who are chained together. At first the two men dislike and distrust each other. However the men are forced to work together in order to survive. By the time the film ends, the men have established a mutual trust and respect.

Racism

Racism in the American health care delivery system is a formidable barrier that strangles transcultural communication between health care professionals and clients. Because the health care profession is regarded as a "caring profession," health care professionals find it difficult to acknowledge that racism exists in the health care workplace. Indeed, for most Euro-American health care professionals, discussions of racism are taboo (Barbee, 1993).

Barbee's article points out that there are three types of racism:

1. *Individual racism:* Individuals are discriminated against because of their visible biological characteristics; for example, black skin or the epicanthic fold of the eyelid in Asians.

2. *Cultural racism:* An individual or institution claims that its cultural heritage is superior to that of other individuals or institutions. For example, during World War II, the Nazis claimed that their Aryan genetic and cultural heritage was superior to the Jewish heritage. They justified persecution of the Jews by convincing themselves that the Jews were an inferior people.

3. *Institutional racism:* Institutions (universities, businesses, hospitals, medical offices) manipulate or tolerate policies that unfairly restrict the opportunities of certain races, cultures, or groups. For example, at one time, black nurses were not allowed to join the American

Nurses Association (ANA). This policy prevented black nurses from having a voice in the regulation of nursing practice and policies.

Because health care professionals perceive themselves as individuals who regard all people as equal, most health care professionals (black and white) will talk about *cultural diversity*, but avoid the word *racism*. Nevertheless, racism exists. For example, in a classic study by Morgan in 1984, researchers found that Euro-American health care students perceived white clients more favorably than black people, and Euro-American clients as more favorable than any other group.

At the institutional level, white students have been admitted more readily to health care programs than black students. Racism is also a factor in the low enrollment numbers of black students in baccalaureate programs compared to 2-year programs. Within the workforce, black health care professionals have complained about not being promoted as readily as white health care professionals (see Chapter 13). Also, black health care professionals have had difficulty publishing in Euro-American professional health journals.

Racism will undermine the health care profession for as long as individuals deny its existence and refuse to talk about it openly and honestly. In the words of Evelyn Barbee (1993):

> One of the flaws in the profession is an unwillingness to recognize that racism is endemic in nursing and health care. This unwillingness results in a lack of discussion about racism and leads to responses that exacerbate the problem.

Bias and Ethnocentrism

Whatever their cultural background, people have a tendency to be **biased** toward their own cultural values, and to feel that their values are *right* and the values of others are *wrong* or *not as good*. Many people are surprised to discover that the values and actions they so admire in their own culture may be looked upon with suspicion by people from other cultures, who are equally biased.

COMMUNICATION CONSIDERATIONS

*The belief that one's own culture or traditions are better than those of other cultures is called **ethnocentrism**. The person who is ethnocentric tends to antagonize and alienate people from other cultures.*

Simultaneous dual ethnocentrism is a component of every health care professional-client relationship. Health care professionals are assessing, judging, evaluating, and reacting to clients on the basis of their own cultural values, medicocentric points of view, and expectations. Simultaneously, clients are using their cultural values to judge and evaluate their health care professional and the Western health care system. As Lydia DeSantis (1994) points out:

> The concept of a simultaneous dual ethnocentrism makes health care professionals keenly aware that they, their patients, their colleagues, and everyone else in the clinical setting are operating under the influence of personal cultural rules, some of which are shared and some of which are not.

Attitudes towards Western medicine constitute one of the biggest barriers to transcultural communication between American health care professionals and clients. American health care professionals tend to be heavily biased toward the Western biomedical health care system because most of them have been educated in this system. Indeed, many health care professionals feel that the biomedical system is the best (and even the only) approach to client care. They may view other health belief systems with suspicion and even contempt, refusing to acknowledge that another approach might have some merit. This ethnocentric attitude can alienate clients from other cultures, who fully believe that *their* therapeutic interventions also have merit. Here is an example of how simultaneous dual ethnocentrism can severely damage the health care professional-client relationship.

> **Example:** Juan Perez, a Mexican immigrant, was hospitalized with a fever of unknown origin. A major conflict developed between the hospital staff and Mr. Perez's family when the family insisted that a *curandero* or folk healer visit the client. When the curandero appeared on the ward with various healing paraphernalia, it was demanded that the healer leave the client's room at once. This so upset Mr. Perez that his family signed him out of the hospital against consent. Had Mr. Perez's health care beliefs been acknowledged he would have been more willing to accept biomedical beliefs.

When white American health care professionals care for people from other cultures, they may be biased not only toward their own health care system, but toward other learned values—such as cleanliness—as well.

> **Example:** During a clinic visit, a Caucasian medical assistant assessed that a Native American child had severe impetigo. The medical assistant observed that the child appeared dirty, and that the mother

had not thoroughly washed her hands. The medical assistant concluded that because the child was dirty, the mother was not taking adequate care of her child.

The medical assistant's assessment was based on a value she learned while studying health promotion, that is, that cleanliness is essential and basic to good health. Her observations translated into a value judgment based on Western bias: "Cleanliness is good. Therefore, a good mother always keeps her child clean."

The mother perceived correctly from the medical assistant's demeanor and tone of voice that this authority figure from the dominant white culture disapproved of her and her parenting skills. She also suspected that the medical assistant was planning to impose her expectations concerning cleanliness and child-rearing.

The Native American mother found herself nodding *yes*, but tuning out the disapproving medical assistant's instructions. The young mother would have been much more inclined to listen had the medical assistant been sensitive in her approach rather than dictatorial. The medical assistant could have said: "I'm sure that you've noticed that your baby has a problem with his skin. When did the problem start? What have you done thus far for the itching? Has it helped? Let's think about this problem together and see what we can do."

By admitting and overcoming her own rigid bias toward cleanliness, the medical assistant would have conveyed that the child needed attention without appearing to judge the mother's standard of cleanliness or her child care skills. As a result, the mother would have been more inclined to listen to the medical assistant and follow through on her suggestions.

COMMUNICATION CONSIDERATIONS

Cultural biases can distort your perception of other people's values and behavior, and thus damage your ability to communicate. To overcome your biases, you must first acknowledge that they exist.

Stereotyping

A cultural **stereotype** is the unsubstantiated assumption that all people of a certain racial and ethnic group are alike. For example: *All Eskimos are* *reserved, deliberate, and noncommittal.* Certainly, some or even the majority of Eskimos may be reserved, deliberate, and noncommittal, but it is cultural stereotyping to state that all Eskimos have these traits. Stereotyping is particularly destructive when negative traits or characteristics are imposed on all members of a cultural group. For example: *All Native Americans are at risk for alcoholism.*

While you must avoid negatively stereotyping clients from different cultural groups, it is nevertheless important to learn about the representative characteristics of different groups. This knowledge will help to smooth and ease your interactions with clients from other cultures.

For example, if you know that Eskimos are raised to be reserved and noncommittal, you will not be offended when Eskimo clients respond to your assessment questions with silence or monosyllables. Conversely, if you are aware that Italian clients tend to be more flamboyant as a group, you will not be surprised when your Italian clients respond to their problems with dramatic gestures and tears.

COMMUNICATION CONSIDERATION

To avoid stereotyping, remember that clients are individuals with unique experiences, and thus may not conform to many (or any) of the characteristics ascribed to their cultural group. Thus, some Eskimos may be outgoing and some Italians may be reserved.

Cultural blind spot syndrome is a form of stereotyping that is a problem for many individuals involved in health care. Cultural blind spot syndrome is the belief that "Just because the client looks and behaves much the way you do, you assume that there are no cultural differences or potential barriers to care" (Buchwald, 1994). For example, white American health care professionals may assume that white American clients believe in the same cultural values as they do. This assumption is false. As you learned in Chapter 2, white Americans come from many different ethnocultural backgrounds—Irish, Russian, German, Jewish, and English to name but a few. In addition, white health care professionals and clients may also belong to different subcultures that have different values. For example, a white male client of Italian descent who is gay will probably have somewhat different values than a white Irish-American individual who is married with 3 children. The negative impact of cultural blind spot syndrome on client care is discussed further in Chapter 10.

Ritualistic Behavior

A ritual is a set procedure for performing a task. In the past, students in health care training were taught to perform their duties in a ritualistic manner. Today, **health care rituals** persist. Many health care rituals are beneficial, such as always performing certain safety checks when preparing and administering medications. However, other rituals, such as always excluding family from the bedside during treatments, are unnecessary and may upset clients and their families. Unfortunately, some health care professionals are so in the habit of performing certain rituals that they become deeply disturbed when these rituals are challenged.

COMMUNICATION CONSIDERATION

As you care for clients, ask yourself which health care rituals are really necessary and which rituals are outdated. If there is no scientific or logical reason to follow a ritual, try to create a new routine that will benefit you and your client.

Language Barriers

Language provides the tools (words) that allow people to express their thoughts and feelings. Thus, language barriers present a grave threat to transcultural communication between health care professionals and clients. There are several types of language barriers that impede communication in the United States. These barriers include:

a. foreign languages,

b. different dialects and regionalisms, and

c. idioms and "street talk."

Foreign Languages, Dialects, and Regionalisms. Even when health care professionals and clients speak the same language, misunderstandings can arise. But when clients come from countries or households where English is *not* the native tongue, the resulting language barrier can bring communication to a halt, producing frustration and conflict.

Unfortunately, it is not possible to be familiar with the hundreds of languages and dialects spoken by clients from different countries and cultures. As noted in Chapter 1, over 6,000 different languages and dialects are spoken today. In addition, the number of people in the United States (all potential clients) who speak languages other than English is growing.

Based on the 1990 census, individuals who spoke languages other than English constituted approximately 10% of the population, or 25 million people. According to a U.S. Education Department report on languages during the 1980s, the number of Spanish speakers increased 65% and speakers of Asian languages rose 98%. The number of people 5 years old and older who spoke languages other than English at home rose approximately 40% (Gannet, 1994). These statistics will be updated in the 2000 census.

Large communities of people who speak languages other than English are flourishing in Southern California, Texas, New Mexico, and Arizona. In Los Angeles alone, over 100 languages other than English are spoken. These languages range from the familiar Spanish tongue to the more exotic language of Gujarati, which is spoken in western India (Compton's, 1995). Moreover, there are many more communities throughout the country where different languages and traditions are common.

As if coping with people who speak different languages is not enough, health care professionals must also be aware that there are hundreds of dialects and regionalisms. Webster's Dictionary defines a **dialect** as the distinctive way a language is spoken or written in a given locality or by a given group of individuals. A **regionalism** is a word, phrase, pronunciation, or custom peculiar to a given region. For example:

- There are three major Chinese dialects: Mandarin, Cantonese, and Shanghainese.

- There are 600 Filipino languages and dialects, among which the most common are Tagalog, Ilocano, Ilonggo, and Cebuano.

- Spanish is not divided into dialects, but there are some regional differences in the use of particular words and phrases. The most recent influx of migrant workers in California speak Mixtec, not Spanish.

- Ebonics, or African-American English, was first discussed in 1975 in *Ebonics: The True Language of Black Folks*, a book by psychology professor Robert L. Williams. Williams derived the word *Ebonics* from *ebony* (for black) and *phonics* for "the scientific study of speech sounds." Williams pointed out that black people are often accused of using bad English when actually they are speaking their own language or dialect, which is based on standard English. In December of 1996, the Oakland School Board in California officially recognized Ebonics as a language or dialect. Concerned that the majority of black students who spoke Ebonics were not doing well in school, the Board passed a resolution calling for improved instruction in standard English (Barnhart and Metcalf, 1997).

To communicate effectively with clients who are not proficient in English, you will need an interpreter. A skilled interpreter can help you, your client, and your client's family overcome the anxiety and frustration produced by language barriers. Chapter 9 describes methods for communicating with clients with limited English proficiency, both with and without an interpreter.

Idioms, Slang, and Street Talk. Sometimes the language barrier—and the type of *interpreter* needed—may not fit the conventional mold just discussed. For example, if you are from a white middle-class background, you may find yourself at a loss to understand the characteristic terms, **idioms**, or expressions used by clients from English-speaking subcultures, be they ghetto blacks, Appalachian hillfolk, or teenagers fluent only in the latest street slang. For example, a health care student from an upper-class background failed to understand the adolescent girls in a clinic until another health care professional explained that *poppers, fizzers,* and *wa-was* referred to prescribed medicines.

Black American speech is particularly rich in idioms. In her book *Black Talk: Words and Phrases From the Hood to the Amen Corner,* Geneva Smitherman (1994) explains that the word *hood* means the neighborhood where a person has grown up and feels comfortable. The phrase *Amen Corner* refers to the corner in a traditional black church where the older church members (usually women) sit. These women, regarded as the *watch dogs of Christ* lead the congregation in Amens.

Some black expressions that you may hear as you work with some black clients in neighborhood clinics or hospitals have the following meanings (Smitherman, 1994):

- *Bad* means excellent or good.
- *BMT* means black man talking. This term is used to express authority.
- *Can't kill nothing and won't nothing die* means having a difficult time.
- *Get on the good foot* means to correct what needs improving.
- *Git out my face* means stop confronting me.
- *Glass house* is a drug house.
- *Come out of a bag* means to behave differently than expected.
- *Hard headed* is a person who refuses to listen to reason.

- *Hoodoo man* is a person skilled in voodoo.

- *The Nation* refers to the Nation of Islam, a black Muslim group.

- *Changes* are personal problems; "He's put me through a lot of changes."

- *Soul* means the essence of life, passion, or emotion.

- *What goes around, come around* is a proverb that expresses the black philosophy that what has happened in the past will occur again, possibly in another form.

Conflicting Perceptions and Expectations

When people from different cultures try to communicate, their best efforts may be thwarted by misunderstandings and even serious conflicts. In health care situations, misunderstandings often arise when the health care professionals and clients have different perceptions and expectations, and consequently misinterpret each others' messages.

Misunderstandings due to cultural differences commonly arise in situations involving food and drink. Imagine that you are taking care of a postoperative Vietnamese female client who, as her culture dictates, is almost constantly attended by her family. You want to clearly instruct family members that they are not to give the client anything to drink. As the family speaks only Vietnamese, you motion that the client is not to drink, and you explain via an interpreter that the client must not drink.

When you return from your lunch break you find your client vomiting, and you observe an empty bowl of soup on her table. Obviously the family has ignored your instructions and fed the client soup. If you angrily say "I told you not to give her anything to drink!" your reaction would be that of many health care professionals in this situation.

However, you later learn from the interpreter that the family knew that they should not give the client water, but they assumed that broth would be beneficial. Vietnamese believe that the sick need to drink broth to rebuild energy. Your intended message (do not drink anything) was not understood by the client's family, and you failed to grasp the family's perception of your instructions (broth is not water, and therefore all right to drink). As a result, the client's family gave her broth and you became frustrated.

COMMUNICATION CONSIDERATION

When there are cultural, behavioral, and language differences between health care professionals, clients, and client's families, there is a greater probability that clients will misunderstand care instructions. To prevent conflicts and misunderstandings, make sure that the message you send the client is the same message that the client receives. When there is a language barrier, you will need to work closely with an interpreter.

Another common area of conflict between health care professionals and clients from diverse cultures involves the perception of health promotion and disease prevention. For example, Hispanics—whose culture is based on honor and pride—may be taught from childhood to bravely accept illness and pain as an inevitable part of human existence. For this reason, traditional Hispanics may see no reason to submit to mammograms or vaccinations (Sabatino, 1993). In the words of the former Surgeon General, Antonia Novello:

> Hispanics are fatalistic. We've been taught that you live, you suffer, you die. That's the way life is. The idea has never been presented that if you take care of your health, if you go to the doctor early, you won't have to suffer pain or discomfort.

Expectations that clients have of health care professionals may also lead to transcultural communication problems. For example, Japanese clients generally look to their family members for the majority of their care, rather than to health care professionals. Even physicians are not in charge; instead they are thought of as *skilled and sympathetic technicians* whose job it is to help families cure the client (Rothenburger, 1990). Health care professionals need to recognize the importance of the Japanese client's family as caregiver, and always communicate with the family before making any important decisions concerning the client's care.

TESTING YOUR KNOWLEDGE

Circle the correct answer.

1. Racism can be classified as
   a. institutional.
   b. individual.
   c. cultural.
   d. all of the above.

2. The belief that one's culture and value system is better than that of another culture is called
   a. bias.
   b. pride.
   c. ethnocentrism.
   d. stereotyping.

3. The statement: "All Asians honor the past" is an example of
   a. ethnocentrism.
   b. stereotyping.
   c. racism.
   d. Cultural Blind Spot Syndrome.

4. Health care professionals who fail to culturally assess a client from the same culture are guilty of
   a. ethnocentrism.
   b. stereotyping.
   c. Cultural Blind Spot Syndrome.
   d. lack of knowledge.

5. Health care professionals who always exclude the client's family from the bedside when giving care are
   a. protective of the patient.
   b. ethnocentric.
   c. ritualistic.
   d. biased.

5

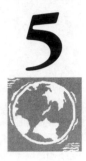

TRANSCULTURAL COMMUNICATION WITHIN THE HEALTH CARE SUBCULTURE

Carol J. Leppa, RN, PhD

KEY TERMS

- Commercial Subculture
- Client Subculture
- Professional Subculture
- Vulnerable Stranger

- Western Biomedical Ethnocentrism
- Western Biomedical Perspective

OBJECTIVES

After completing this chapter, you should be able to:

- Discuss cultural values, beliefs, and behaviors of the Western health care system.
- Describe potential communication conflicts among health care providers, management, and clients within the hospital environment.
- Describe the health care subculture and its development.
- Discuss the perspective of the client in the hospital environment.
- Identify three strategies to help you recognize and deal with Western health care ethnocentrism in the hospital setting.

INTRODUCTION

Learning about culture requires learning about yourself. It is often easier and more interesting to learn about cultural beliefs and practices that are exotic or different from your own. However, to develop a true appreciation for the power of culture, it is necessary to learn about how our own culture affects our beliefs, our actions, and our expectations. This is imperative in the health care profession where there are multiple layers and overlaps in a variety of cultural and subcultural groups. Understanding these layers and overlapping loyalties and beliefs will help you to identify communication problems and illuminate potential solutions.

This chapter explores the concept of transcultural communication within the subculture of the Western health care system. It explores the overlapping subcultures within the health care system, and identifies specific areas where miscommunications can occur due to cultural differences. By understanding the perspectives of professional, business, and client subcultures, health care professionals working within their professional subculture will learn how to broker communications within and among these varied groups.

WESTERN HEALTH CARE SYSTEM SUBCULTURE

The Western health care system includes all individuals and organizations involved in the education, professional practice, delivery, business, and consumption of health care in what is called Western Culture. The Western health care system is a subculture of white Western Culture. The white Western culture and its tradition promotes an almost exclusive belief in and reliance on the biomedical belief system.

Members of this tradition value *technology* almost exclusively in the struggle to conquer disease. Western health care professionals gather enormous amounts of data (laboratory tests, invasive procedures, x-rays, body scans, review of systems) in order to diagnosis and treat the underlying pathophysiology. Their goal is to rapidly resolve the client's symptoms with biomedical interventions, and ultimately cure the pathology. Although some elements of the popular and traditional/folk sectors of health care have gained credence within Western health care (including the recent recognition of a variety of alternative or complementary health practices), the dominant belief system remains biomedical.

The strong, shared belief in the biomedical approach to health care has sometimes resulted in **Western biomedical ethnocentrism**—a serious barrier to communication. This ethnocentrism is displayed in the derision that greets client use of or provider interest in alternative health practices. Even the term *alternative* indicates that these practices are outside of the accepted biomedical practices, and thus will be tolerated only if they do not interfere with the *real* biomedical treatment plan. Interest in alternative (more recently called *complimentary*) therapies has increased, and research on these remedies has been funded by the National Institutes of Health. Nevertheless, clients and professionals who are interested in, use, or practice these therapies may find it difficult to communicate with professionals who work within the strongly biomedical culture of Western health care.

COMMUNICATION CONSIDERATIONS

 The strong biomedical culture of the Western health care system may result in communication problems between professionals and clients who choose to use alternative or complimentary therapies.

While the Western health care system is a subculture of its own, it is also a multifaceted collection of other identifiable subcultural groups. The goals of diagnosis and treatment using biomedical methods are shared in varying degrees in the specialized health care settings of private physician or nurse practitioner offices, hospitals, clinics, home care, rehabilitation, and long-term care facilities. The goals change somewhat in long-term care facilities and hospice, yet they are still strongly connected with the Western health care system values, beliefs, and behaviors.

The hospital is the most visible and well known of the subcultural settings of Western health care, due in large part to the use of hospital settings in popular television programs. The hospital setting is a microcosm of the Western health care system, and an excellent place to explore the issues of transcultural communication within Western health care.

HOSPITAL SUBCULTURE

The hospital in Western culture is a complex organization dedicated to the common goal of health care delivery. *Health* is generally understood to be the absence, minimization, or control of disease processes. The hospital is a complex organization with multiple players involved in a variety of hierarchical relationships founded on the goal of health care delivery. The varied players in the organization may work in concert or in conflict depending on the cultural expectations that they bring to this environment.

PROFESSIONAL SUBCULTURE

One of the major subcultures operating within the hospital and the health care delivery system in general is the **professional subculture** of the direct care providers. This professional subculture includes nurses, physicians, therapists, and pharmacists. These practitioners are licensed to provide health care by legislative authority. Although each of these professional groups has a strong subgroup identity and subculture, they share in the professional health care values of beneficence and non-maleficence (being of benefit and doing no harm) established in the Hippocratic oath.

Professional groups have codes of conduct that define appropriate behavior including veracity (telling the truth), fidelity (loyalty and keeping promises), and professional and client confidentiality. Western health care professionals also embrace the value of individual autonomy that is a major part of white Western culture as discussed in Chapter Two.

COMMUNICATION CONSIDERATIONS

 The practice of informed consent and client rights is based on the value of individual autonomy. The Patients' Bill of Rights is prominently displayed in Western hospitals.

Members of the professional subculture in the Western health care system strongly support the value of being a benefit to clients, and they have been educated to put the client first, largely without regard to the financial costs or effective use of resources. Professionals focus on their relationships with individual clients, and the accurate biomedical diagnosis and treatment. They have taken an oath and are licensed to help clients, and this guides their behaviors and communications.

COMMERCIAL OR BUSINESS SUBCULTURE

The **commercial** (or business) **subculture** is another strong subculture in the Western health care system. For example, as complex organizations, hospitals need expert business managers and administrators who can maintain an environment for meeting the goal of delivering health care. The values that members of the business subculture bring to the hospital environment include maintaining the health of the organization through support systems (supplies, building maintenance), financial responsibility (paying employees, collecting payments), and market competition. The language of *fiscal responsibility, the bottom line, outcomes-based care,* and the increasingly popular *managed care* provides external evidence of the business culture in health care.

COMMUNICATION PROBLEMS BETWEEN SUBCULTURES

All health care settings need competent and dedicated administrators and managers from the business culture to provide the environment for health care delivery. All health care settings also need competent and dedicated care providers from the professional subculture. When these cultures clash, communication conflicts result, producing disagreements about cost-effective care. Professional care providers tend to focus on effective care based on the biomedical belief system—is the pathology corrected or mitigated? Managers and administrators ask difficult questions about the monetary value or worth of a treatment, and the cost–benefit analysis of the health outcome. Discussions that argue these points are strongly based in the cultural beliefs of the participants.

Bringing cost into a treatment decision is strongly counter to the professional cultural ethic. For example, to eliminate mild or moderate chest pain, physicians may advocate coronary artery bypass surgery for single-vessel heart disease as the best option, even though surgery is more expensive than other interventions. Ignoring the costs of treatments is strongly counter to the responsible business ethic. From a business perspective, a cost–benefits analysis of surgery versus the less expensive medical management is central to making a treatment decision. Knowing that there are professional/administrative cultural issues involved in discussions helps all parties reach better compromises and solutions (McArthur & Moore, 1997).

OTHER HEALTH CARE SUBCULTURES

There are other important subcultures in Western Health Care related to and yet significantly different from the hospital subculture. These subcultures include the areas of long-term care and community-based health care. Although these subcultures are affiliated with the hospital, they have their own guiding values and beliefs. Communication problems may arise when professionals from these subcultures interact with hospital-based professionals. For example, the long-term care subculture encompasses a wider range of *successful outcomes* than the control of pathophysiology of disease processes, and includes expected progressive decline and death. Clients are called *residents* to reflect the combination of home and health care environments. Professionals who move from the acute care to the long-term care environment frequently experience a culture shock as they learn new behaviors and expectations for professional care.

Community-based health care environments include a wide variety of settings; for example, hospice, home-care, public health clinics, ambulatory care, and school health. Each of these settings combines Western health care values with the values that guide the particular setting.

Practicing Within the Health Care Subculture

While specific behaviors may differ from hospital to hospital and setting to setting, health care professionals who form the health care subculture share many values, beliefs, behaviors, and rituals. The health care subculture in turn overlaps, has commonalties with, and also conflicts with the hospital subculture, the professional subculture, and the dominant American culture. Health care professionals in long-term care and community-based health care environments have similar overlaps and conflicts.

The use of technology is a major part of the health care environment, with higher status attributed to those professionals who work in the high technology environments of Intensive Care and Emergency Departments. It is no accident that these are the environments that are portrayed on popular television programs; they reflect the Western cultural value of conquering or mastering the biomedical disease enemy—preferably using state-of-the-art technology.

The professional subculture shares the professional ethic of beneficence and a relative dislike for or distrust of the concern with the costs or business side of client care. This can result in difficult and frustrating communications with managers and administrators. Health care professionals must learn the language and values of both the professional and business subcultures.

The Health Care Subculture and Language

Health care is defined as a culture because it is learned in schools, shared across multiple health care environments, and transmitted from one generation of professionals to the next. Health care professionals follow rules of behavior that are both specific to a particular health care environment and generalized to a specific profession. Whether defined as a culture or a subculture, health care has a distinct identity, value system, and expected behaviors (Suominen et al., 1997). One of these expected behaviors is *language*.

Health care professionals use professional biomedical language on the job and readily converse with other health care professionals in terms often incomprehensible to people not employed in health care. Some of this language is shared by all health care professionals; for example, terms relating to pathophysiology, diagnostic tests, and treatments. Other language is specific to particular environments (e.g., the operating room) where personnel use special terms which can be incomprehensible to health care professionals from other areas. Although the specialty-specific dialects may cause minor communication problems between care providers, these problems may become major for clients and their families who struggle to understand. The language of Western health care is English, which can add to communication problems with non-native English health care workers and clients (see Chapter 13).

Example: This problem is reflected in my experience with a specialty dialect when I first worked on a cardiac medical–surgical unit. The first day I listened to morning report, I heard about the client who was a "cabbage times three"—which I later learned referred to the client with a three-vessel coronary bypass graft (or *CABGx3* in the surgical notes). This dialect was not covered in my education or in my hospital orientation, and I can only wonder what non-health care workers would make of being described as a "cabbage times three!"

THE CLIENT SUBCULTURE

As mentioned in Chapter 2, clients in hospitals and other health care settings also form a distinct subculture. Whatever their culture of origin, professional or occupational subculture, adopted cultural identity, degree of assimilation or acculturation to Western culture, or religious identity, clients all become members of a distinct **client subculture** when treated in the hospital setting.

Because the language of health care is unique and the schedules of daily activities are new, every client enters this hospital environment as a **vulnerable stranger** in need of care (Toumishey, 1989). Repeated treatment in hospitals produces some clients who become more or less acculturated to the hospital culture. However, even these clients remain vulnerable with each hospital admission, because when clients enter the hospital they become isolated from their usual life routines.

Example: On being ordered to take his clothes off for examination, a newly-admitted client explained this revelation:

This incident, trivial in itself, brought two points home to me in immediate succession. To start with, my own individuality, my own independence, my private self and what it meant to me, had, as though by her telling remark, been taken away from me. Until a couple of hours ago, outside the hospital environment, I had been a free agent, free in so far as it is possible to choose, free to determine, and free to exercise my own will on matters large and small. But in the hospital I felt entrapped. I had entered a new environment, a new culture, which had its own established rules and norms. I was now expected to learn and follow the rules of the new culture—in other words play the role of patient (Laungani, 1992, p.10).

This client, a psychology professor who had conducted research in many hospital environments, now found himself a stranger in the health care environment.

Laungani describes his three-month hospitalization and how he had to learn to survive in this relatively unfamiliar (to him) culture in a new and unfamiliar role. He emphasizes how clients are expected to be compliant and grateful. He also discusses how the nature of being dependent and vulnerable interplay with learning how to behave as a good client and fit in, so that he could get the help he so desperately needed. Toumishey (1989) describes how vulnerable strangers (such as Professor Laungani) must determine an appropriate new role, the accepted meanings of behavior in the new environment, expectations of others, and methods of coping. This is difficult enough for clients who are familiar with the Western health care culture, as Professor Laungani certainly was. It is far more difficult for those unfamiliar with or from a radically different cultural background.

When clients become *residents* in long-term care facilities they face additional challenges. Now the subculture encourages a *home-like* environment yet this is frequently overshadowed by the needs of the community of residents. Home-like is no longer an individual personal space, a primary value in Western culture, but a shared living space (frequently intimately shared) with continued and increasing dependency on caregivers for daily needs. Caregivers and residents become a close community/family with extended relationships, which may be enjoyable or difficult and may continue day after day. In addition, the personal cultures of the caregivers may radically conflict with those of the residents.

HEALTH CARE PROFESSIONALS AS CULTURE BROKERS BETWEEN SUBCULTURES

Health care professionals work within and through all of these Western Health Care subcultures. Health care professionals need to be aware of their own subculture as well as the values and associated behaviors of the other subcultures to be effective in holistic client care delivery and client advocacy.

In order to participate effectively in transcultural communications in the hospital environment, you need to evaluate your own beliefs, biases, and behaviors. Self-assessment exercises help with this evaluation. In addition to these, study your work environment from the perspective of culture. What are the rituals that you observe and participate in? What are the patterns of movement, daily routines, clothing, equipment, and language that are essential elements of your work? These elements express the cultural values of the **Western biomedical perspective**—efficiency, timeliness, technology, and science/pathophysiology. You will continue to be a part of this culture of health care, but you will be sensitized to the wider meaning of your beliefs and actions.

Try to see your work environment as a stranger (client) would. One method of doing this is to experience the role of the stranger. Visit an environment where you do not know the language or accepted behaviors. Attend a public event in a neighborhood where you are in the minority. Attend a religious service of which you have no previous knowledge or experience. Any of these experiences will help you understand the feeling of being a stranger.

Observe yourself and your colleagues for signs of ethnocentric reactions—shock, anger, laughter—when confronted with beliefs and behaviors that conflict with the world view of Western biomedicine. Although surprise may be a common part of contact with different health care beliefs and practices, as a professional you need to demonstrate respect. As discussed in other parts of this book, a successful transcultural communication requires that health care professionals show respect and work with clients to understand their health care needs and beliefs. Remember that your own biomedical belief system may seem odd or silly to the client. To work toward a successful and mutually acceptable negotiated treatment plan, explore how your Western beliefs fit and/or conflict with the client's beliefs.

Brokering Between Clients and the Health Care Subculture

Health care professionals are in a vital position for negotiating the interface between the client culture and the Western health care culture. There are three steps basic to this brokering:

1. Be aware of the fact that the Western health care system is a culture of its own with rituals and language often incomprehensible to clients.

2. Carefully explore the client's cultural background and needs.

3. Explore and explain the particular client subculture to which the client has been admitted.

An awareness of the potential confusion and conflicts among these three subcultures is necessary for health care professionals to function as both client advocate and professional health care provider. Health care professionals can effectively translate the complexities of health care to clients, as well as translating the client's values and beliefs to other Western health care providers.

Brokering Between Professional Subcultures

Health care professionals must work with a variety of personnel in Western health care and can become proficient in communicating in a variety of situations. For example, professionals faced with explaining the use of alternative (complimentary) therapies to colleagues in the Western biomedical system would be wise to explore these therapies in an open and interested manner. It is also important to share research on the use and success of the therapies with colleagues in a non-threatening manner. The standard research approach for testing the efficacy of therapeutic touch provides an excellent example. There are a number of articles on the use of therapeutic touch in a variety of health care settings (Daley, 1997; Easter, 1997; Fryback & Reinert, 1997; Kotora, 1997; Snyder, 1997). When selecting references to share with Western practitioner colleagues, include articles from the more mainstream and accepted biomedical perspective as well as newer, alternative publications. Those health care professionals skeptical of alternative health care practices should familiarize themselves with this literature because clients often use a variety of alternative (complementary) treatments.

COMMUNICATION CONSIDERATIONS

Understanding the various subcultural groups in Western health care is the first step in effective communications. Exploring these groups and their interactions and conflicts will increase effectiveness as a health care professional. Learning how to translate and broker communications among the various groups will help avoid the frustrations of miscommunications and potential problems.

TESTING YOUR KNOWLEDGE

Circle the correct answer.

1. What type of transcultural communication conflict may occur when a professional and an administrator disagree over the need for and cost of increased staffing?
   a. hospital subculture conflict
   b. professional subculture conflict
   c. client subculture conflict
   d. Western biomedical culture conflict

2. What type of transcultural communication conflict may occur when a medical assistant changes jobs to a new unit in the same hospital?
   a. hospital subculture conflict
   b. professional subculture conflict
   c. client subculture conflict
   d. Western biomedical culture conflict

3. What type of transcultural communication conflict may occur when a physician angrily refuses to consider the use of therapeutic touch in post-op client care?
   a. hospital subculture conflict
   b. professional subculture conflict
   c. client subculture conflict
   d. Western biomedical culture conflict

4. Which Western health care system subculture has vulnerability and dependence as primary characteristics?
   a. hospital subculture
   b. business subculture
   c. client subculture
   d. professional subculture

5. When is *culture shock* likely to occur among health care subcultures?
   a. beginning a first job after graduation
   b. moving from one job to another
   c. a professional becomes a client in the health care system
   d. all of the above

6. What are common expressions of an ethnocentric reaction to therapy?
   a. believing in multiple methods of appropriate care
   b. use of therapeutic touch to treat post-op pain
   c. non-compliance with prescribed treatment
   d. laughter, anger and/or shock when encountering a therapy that is new or different

UNIT ONE
EVALUATION

EVALUATING YOUR TRANSCULTURAL COMMUNICATION GOALS AND BASIC KNOWLEDGE

The following exercises highlight some of the concepts discussed in earlier sections. Make a note if you are selecting a different option than you would have *prior* to studying Unit I.

Exercise One: Altering Transcultural Communication Approaches

After reading the chapters in Unit I, answer these questions as honestly as possible.

1. What are your major transcultural communication goals?

   _____

   _____

   _____

   _____

2. What factors *in yourself might support* your goals?
   a. _____
   b. _____
   c. _____

3. What factors in your *clinical setting might support* your goals?
   a. _____
   b. _____
   c. _____

4. What factors in *yourself might hinder* your goals?
   a. _____
   b. _____
   c. _____

5. What factors in your *clinical setting might hinder* your goals?
   a. _____
   b. _____
   c. _____

6. In what ways would you like to alter or improve your transcultural communication style or approach?

_____

_____

Exercise Two: Reviewing Your Transcultural Interaction Diary

1. Have you had any positive interactions with clients from other races or cultures? _____

   What did you learn about each client's cultural values and beliefs?

   _____

   _____

   What communication style (verbal and nonverbal) did each client use?

   _____

   _____

   How did you respond to each client's communication style?

   _____

   _____

2. Have you had any *difficult or unsuccessful interactions* with clients from other cultures?

   _____

   _____

   Which transcultural communication *stumbling block* do you feel was instrumental in creating a negative interaction?

   _____

   _____

   Are you aware of any other stumbling blocks such as bias, stereotyping, or ritualistic behavior that could damage your transcultural interactions?

   _____

   _____

3. Chapter 5, *Transcultural Communication Within the Health Care Subculture*, suggests that you visit an environment where you do not know the language or social customs. How did you feel about this experience?

   _____

   _____

   What did you learn from this experience that you can apply to your work with people from other cultures?

   _____

   _____

Exercise Three: Evaluating Your Readiness for Unit II, Developing Your Transcultural Communication Skills

Write a brief response to these questions, which are drawn from topics discussed in Chapters 1 through 5.

1. What is the objective of communication in the health care setting?

   _____

   _____

2. What is communication competence?

   _____

   _____

   On a scale from 1 to 10 (10 being the most competent) how competently do you communicate with clients from other cultures?

   _____

   _____

3. Give four reasons why it is currently so important for health care professionals to learn transcultural communication skills.

   a. _____

   b. _____

   c. _____

   d. _____

4. Cultural values are principles or standards that members of a cultural group share in common. Values serve at least seven important functions:

   a. _____

   b. _____

   c. _____

   d. _____

   e. _____

   f. _____

   g. _____

   What cultural values do you believe in?

   _____

   What subcultures do you belong to?

   _____

   What subcultural values do you believe in?

   _____

5. What are the three major health belief systems?

a. _____

b. _____

c. _____

Do you accept the health beliefs of clients who are from other cultures?

_____

Why or why not? _____

_____

6. What are the four major health care systems?

a. _____

b. _____

c. _____

d. _____

What experiences have you had with each health care system?

_____

_____

7. What factors determine a person's response to illness?

_____

_____

_____

What do you feel is acceptable behavior for a hospitalized client?

_____

_____

8. Each culture has different standards for *verbal* communication. Give transcultural examples of the following:

a. Word choice: _____

b. Emotional expressiveness and volume: _____

c. Voice inflection: _____

d. Directness: _____

e. Use of silence: _____

9. *Nonverbal communication* also differs from culture to culture. Give examples of different types of nonverbal communication.

a. _____

b. _____

c. _____

d. _____

e. _____

10. According to Rothenburger, what are the seven stages that people pass through during their initial encounters with individuals from different cultures?

    a. _____

    b. _____

    c. _____

    d. _____

    e. _____

    f. _____

    g. _____

    What stages have you experienced when developing relationships with people from other cultures?

    _____

    _____

11. What is simultaneous dual ethnocentrism, and how does it affect every professional–client relationship?

    _____

    _____

12. In what ways do language barriers present a grave threat to communication between health care professionals and clients?

    _____

    _____

    What different types of language barriers have you encountered in the clinical area?

    _____

    _____

    _____

13. What are the four different types of transcultural conflicts that can occur within the health care subculture? Give an example of each.

    a. _____

    b. _____

    c. _____

    d. _____

    What types of transcultural conflicts have you experienced in the clinical area?

    _____

    _____

UNIT TWO

DEVELOPING TRANSCULTURAL COMMUNICATION SKILLS

UNIT TWO
ASSESSMENT

ASSESSING YOUR TRANSCULTURAL
COMMUNICATION SKILLS

Exercise One: Assessing How Comfortable You Feel When Communicating With Clients From Other Cultures

As you communicate with people from other cultures, you will gradually become more comfortable during transcultural interactions. The more comfortable you feel, the more comfortable your clients will feel. Exercise One will help you assess your current level of comfort with transcultural interactions. The statements that follow contain assignments that you might receive in the clinical area or community. Using the following 5 levels of comfort, rate how you feel about performing each assignment.

- Level 1: I feel very uncomfortable.
- Level 2: I feel rather uncomfortable.
- Level 3: I feel fairly comfortable.
- Level 4: I feel comfortable.
- Level 5: I feel very comfortable.

1. *Assignment:* Go into a market in an ethnic neighborhood and ask the store personnel about the different foods that are available, and how to prepare them. **1 2 3 4 5**

2. *Assignment:* Go to an ethnic pharmacy and speak with the pharmacist about which over-the-counter drugs the people in the neighbor tend to purchase. **1 2 3 4 5**

3. *Assignment:* Visit a cuandero or folk healer and learn about the various healing modalities that he or she uses. **1 2 3 4 5**

4. *Assignment:* Assess an older Asian female client who is accompanied by many concerned, attentive family members. **1 2 3 4 5**

5. *Assignment:* Assess an Italian client who is constantly crying and grabbing onto your hand. **1 2 3 4 5**

6. *Assignment:* Provide home care to a 4-month-old child whose mother has placed open scissors (resembling a cross) under the child's pillow in order to ward off evil spirits. **1 2 3 4 5**

7. *Assignment:* Give a complete bath to a Vietnamese woman with the husband and older children present throughout the procedure.

1 2 3 4 5

8. *Assignment:* Have a medical interpreter help you collect verbal data from a client who does not speak English. **1 2 3 4 5**

9. *Assignment:* Assess a client who does not speak English without the help of an interpreter. **1 2 3 4 5**

Exercise Two: Assessing Your Point of View Toward Transcultural Situations

What is your attitude toward transcultural situations? Do you feel that it is very important to consider the client's cultural background when giving care? Or do you feel that cultural considerations are much less important than other aspects of care? Select the one answer that best describes your point of view *now*, before you proceed with the chapters in this unit. There is no scoring for these questions.

1. The health care professional when interacting with clients needs to
   a. elicit the client's perspective about being ill.
   b. share food with the client.
   c. adopt the client's customs.
   d. efficiently manage the care of the client.

2. A culturally sensitive health care professional
   a. is knowledgeable about cultural traits.
   b. adheres to institutional regulations.
   c. adapts communication style to be congruent with the client's expectations.
   d. develops expertise in asking questions to gather client data.

3. The attention that should be allotted to communication in transcultural settings is
   a. little or none as few instances are truly cultural exchanges.
   b. fairly significant because more clients are from diverse cultural backgrounds.
   c. only of consequence in some settings.
   d. extremely important and necessary for holistic care.

4. When working with a client in the emergency room who has limited English proficiency, I would
   a. have a close family member interpret for the client.
   b. rely on a telephone language service for pertinent information.
   c. make an effort to find a qualified interpreter.
   d. attempt to communicate with the client using a phrase chart.

5. When interacting with clients I would
   a. encourage them to express their views of illness.
   b. discourage personal beliefs as they have little connection to the health care plan.
   c. elicit information about their family.
   d. insist that they need to comply with their care plan for their own good.

Exercise Three: Using Your *Transcultural Interaction Diary*

1. In Unit One you set up your *Transcultural Interaction Diary*. To help you apply the principles that you will learn in Unit II, record any positive or negative transcultural transactions that involve (a) acting as a participant observer in an ethnic community, (b) establishing communication with a client from another culture; (c) overcoming transcultural communication barriers; and (d) working with and without an interpreter.

2. You may want to write some of your diary entries in the form of a *process recording*. A process recording (or a verbatim report) is a written record in which you record every word that you and the client exchange within a certain time period. Process recordings should also contain your observations of the client's nonverbal communication. Although different formats may be used for process recording, many people like to record their data in 3 columns—one for the client's words, one for your words, and one for an analysis of the conversation or personal notes.

3. As you study this unit, try to implement the various transcultural communication techniques suggested in the chapters, and record how using these techniques helped you to communicate better with your clients.

4. You may also want to concentrate on overcoming one transcultural communication barrier each week. For example, during one week you might decide to focus on *stereotyping*. Recall from Chapter 4 that a cultural stereotype is the unsubstantiated assumption that all people of a certain race or ethnic group are alike. Here are two possible diary entries.

Week of March 18th: Watch Out For Stereotyping

3/18 Today, I was assigned a Jewish client, and I caught myself thinking that I didn't want to take care of this woman because *all* Jewish clients are very demanding, and her demands were going to interfere with my other client assignments. I immediately realized that I was making a false assumption. Actually, the client turned out to be very pleasant and cooperative.

3/21 While I was eating in the hospital cafeteria, a coworker remarked that *all* Mexicans eat a lot of fatty foods. He said that refried beans cooked in lard is a daily staple. I said that wasn't true. I told the coworker that I had recently spent some time as a participant–observer in a Mexican community, and I found that *some* Mexicans ate a lot of fatty foods, but many others were watching their fat intake.

5. Remember to keep your diary in a private place. You will not feel as free to write about your transcultural interactions if other people might read your personal thoughts, feelings, and experiences.

6

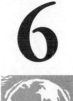

EXPLORING TRANSCULTURAL COMMUNICATION AS A PARTICIPANT-OBSERVER

Lydia DeSantis, PhD, RN, FAAN

KEY TERMS

- Context
- Ethnography
- Explicit Awareness
- Fieldwork
- Grand Tour Questions
- Key Informants

- Participant–Observation
- Rapid Assessment Procedures (RAP)
- Repetitive Social Situations
- Selective Inattention
- Sensory Overload

OBJECTIVES

After completing this chapter, you should be able to:

- Define the components of a repetitive social situation.
- Identify the four phases of participant–observation.
- Define the characteristics of each phase of participant–observation.
- Discuss the meaning of being an insider and outsider in participant–observation.
- Describe the characteristics of a good key informant.

INTRODUCTION

Health care professionals, like all human beings, are continually engaged in the process of observation. We observe something every second of our conscious lives, and process a tremendous amount of information at various levels of awareness. Information remains in our conscious awareness (**explicit awareness**) when we use it to make sense of social situations and to participate in them appropriately.

Through the process of **selective inattention**, information not needed to function appropriately in the immediate environment is sifted out and falls by the cognitive wayside. We just tune it out by not consciously acknowledging it. Selective inattention helps us avoid **sensory overload**, or the inability to process and cope with all of the environmental stimuli we receive (Spradley, 1980). Selective inattention allows health care professionals to give an injection without noting how far away the chair is from the bed, seeing the title of what the client is reading, noting what color the room is painted, or identifying what is playing on the television. All of those things are present or happening, but they remain out of the health care professional's explicit awareness because they are of no consequence to the task at hand.

REPETITIVE SOCIAL SITUATIONS

We learn the verbal and nonverbal behavior expected of us through our observation and participation in **repetitive social situations (RSS)**, or everyday events that occur over and over again. Repetitive social situations are comprised of time, place, person(s), activities, and their interactions (Spradley, 1980). They recur across time with the same or similar types of individuals and in the same or similar kinds of places (settings). Observation and participation in RSSs helps us learn the cognitive maps (cultural rules for and patterns of behavior expected of us) that allow us to conduct our daily lives, relate to others, and provide care with a minimum of misunderstanding, confusion, or conflict.

When some aspect of an RSS changes or is unfamiliar, those involved may become confused, uncomfortable, anxious, angry, hostile, or unable to function. More commonly, their selective inattention may prevent them from even realizing a change has occurred; cause them to dismiss it as inconsequential; consider it a misunderstanding, mistake, or ignorance on the part of another; or simply demand that the other person(s) conform to the way things ought to be, do the right thing, or act properly.

Interactions with clients are types of RSSs. Health care professionals are most comfortable when interacting with clients who share their understanding of what behaviors are expected and act accordingly. When changes occur in some aspect of the usual client interaction, professionals and clients may experience discomfort, anxiety, and anger because their expectations of each other have not been met or they have been unable to relate to one another in the usual and heretofore appropriate manner. Our discomfort becomes more pronounced when we must function in a different care setting, such as in clients' homes, neighborhood clinics, or mobile vans. Our selective inattention often causes us to miss important verbal and nonverbal cues in altered or new social situations. These cues can help us identify the rules and patterns of communication behavior in the new setting if we are aware of them.

CONTEXT

All RSSs occur in a **context**. Context is the temporal, social, cultural, physical, chemical, biological, and metaphysical environments in which we live, and which affects our everyday existence, adaptation, and interaction.

Due to the ever-changing temporal and/or other aspects of natural settings, contexts are never precisely identical. For example, RSSs occur at different times of the day, week, or year; additional people are present; placement of furniture or equipment varies; the temperature is warmer or colder; or client needs are different. The ever-changing nature of the context in which RSSs occur requires that all behavior be contextualized; that is, behavior is viewed and analyzed based on the who, what, when, where, and why of the RSS. Contextualizing behavior helps health care professionals to overcome their selective inattention in RSSs, and better understand and adapt to the cultural rules for and patterns of behavior that govern their client interactions.

COMMUNICATION CONSIDERATIONS

When observing the dynamics of health care professionals-client encounters, we need to be like "investigative reporters" and gather information on the who, what, where, and when of the interaction. Who is present? What is happening? Where is it happening? When is it happening? Information from the "Five Ws" will help us understand the "sixth W"—the why (meaning) of the event. Why is it happening? Once we get the facts of the story together, we will better understand the cultural rules for and patterns of behavior expected of us when we interact with clients..

Because client populations are becoming more culturally diverse and the health care environment and modes of care delivery are rapidly changing, we need to develop methods of overcoming selective inattention in order to learn about the cultural beliefs and practices of the populations we serve and the settings in which we practice. It is impossible to learn everything about every cultural group in existence or the variations within each group or RSS. However, we can use modified forms of the anthropological method of **participant-observation** (PO) to overcome our selective inattention, contextualize behavior, and gain a relatively rapid understanding of different groups, settings, cultural beliefs and practices, and modes of communication.

PARTICIPANT-OBSERVATION

One of the best ways to learn about cultural groups is to observe and interact (participate) with them as they go about their daily lives. We do this naturally when we vacation in other countries, attend ethnic wedding and birthday celebrations, or just sit and talk about life with friends from different ethnic groups. All of these activities help us to better understand and communicate during client encounters.

COMMUNICATION CONSIDERATIONS

Learning about multiple aspects of the culture of various ethnic groups is important. Culture is an integrated system of values, beliefs, and practices that stems from a common world view (concept of reality). Culture guides decision making and behavior in all dimensions of life. As you expand your cultural knowledge about a group, you will also enhance your understanding of the beliefs and practices guiding their health behavior.

Everyday Observation and Participant-Observation

Health care professionals, like all human beings, are participants and observers in the realities of their daily existence. However, there are distinct differences between being an ordinary participant in an RSS and being a participant-observer in the anthropological sense (Spradley, 1979, 1980). For example, participant–observers at a well-baby clinic would do the following:

Action	Example
Enter RSS with two objectives: (a) to actively and appropriately engage in the events occurring, and (b) to consciously observe the who, what, where, when, and why.	
Seek to overcome their selective inattention and become explicitly aware of information they normally block out.	What are mothers doing while waiting to be seen at well-baby clinics? How does the context affect their behavior?
Use *wide angle lenses*, that is, pay particular attention to (take mental pictures of) all that is occurring in RSS, and not just focus on what is necessary to accomplish immediate tasks.	Who is present and what is happening at the well-baby clinic while the mothers are waiting to be seen?
Experience how it is to *be both an insider and outsider at the same time* in RSS.	How do my colleagues and the mothers respond to each others' verbal and nonverbal behavior when they interact? Who initiates the interaction? When and where does it occur? What tone of voice do the staff and mothers use? Does the health care professionals' verbal and non-verbal behavior change when there is too little time and too many mothers and infants to see and teach? Do health care professionals behave differently with mothers from different racial, ethnic, and socio-economic groups? What happens when I interact with the mothers? Do I act, speak, and feel the same way as my colleagues?

	Did I behave as a culturally sensitive professional?
Be more *introspective* and use themselves as the *data gathering instrument* to: (a) determine and understand the cultural rules for and patterns of behavior and (b) gain skill in following those rules by behaving like an insider (native).	Why did I act, say, and feel as I did when I did? Did I behave as the mothers expected me to behave? Did the mothers respond to my behavior like I thought they would?
Interview persons (**key informants**) who are participants in the RSS or others who are experts in client–staff behavior who can tell you what is occurring and why.	Before I leave, I want to talk to some of the health care professionals and mothers to learn what and why they did, said, or felt during the RSS that I observed. Were they doing, saying, and feeling the same things as I thought based on my observations? What do I need to know to feel more comfortable and to be more effective? How can I get the mothers to ask more questions?
Keep *fieldnotes* (written records) of their objective (what they observe) and subjective observations (what they see, feel, and do) in the RSS. Fieldnotes help to reconstruct and contextualize experiences at a later time.	When I look back over my first month as a participant–observer in the well-baby clinic, do I feel and act differently now than after the first week? What happened to affect my behavior and feelings? Am I more comfortable and better able to interact with and teach the mothers now? Why is this? When and why did my comfort level change? Are the mothers more willing to listen and respond to me?

In the traditional anthropological method of PO, the anthropologist conducts **fieldwork** (studying and living with a group) for a year or more preparatory to writing an **ethnography**, a description and analysis of a group's culture. Health care professionals cannot realistically take a year or more to learn the cultural rules for and patterns of behaviors of all of the groups with which they interact. However, aspects of two types of PO can be combined to help us understand how to obtain cultural knowledge about ethnic groups and the settings where we provide care. The traditional four-stage PO process will serve as the framework for the discussion. **Rapid assessment procedures** (RAP), a modified or short-hand version of PO, will be used to demonstrate how health care professionals can quickly gather information about specific, circumscribed aspects of their clients' cultural beliefs and practices that affect their health (Scrimshaw & Hurtado, 1987).

Phases of Participant–Observation

The four phases of the traditional PO process are:

1. complete observer
2. observer-as-participant
3. participant-as-observer
4. complete participant.

Participant–observation is actually a continuum that participant-observers go back and forth on, depending on the nature of the RSS, and the depth of their understanding of the cultural rules governing the behavior of those in the RSS. When on the *observation* portion of the continuum, participant–observers are better able to stand aside, see the interactions in the RSS more completely and objectively, and validate information provided by key informants. For example, dietitians who observe their colleagues teaching diabetic clients can better evaluate the effectiveness of teaching–learning techniques by using their wide angle lenses to observe the interactions of their colleagues and clients rather than by doing the teaching themselves. By not actively engaging in the teaching–learning process as insiders, their selective inattention and personal investment in the success of the teaching endeavor are lessened. They can focus more on how aspects of the context affect the teaching–learning process as it unfolds; observe how verbal and nonverbal behaviors of health care professionals and clients affect their interactions; and talk with participants afterward about their perceptions of the session.

When on the *participation* portion of the continuum, participant–observers can subjectively experience as insiders what those in the RSS are experiencing.

They can simultaneously understand the experience from the other persons' points of view, and raise additional questions for further PO and confirmation of new cultural knowledge and skills. For instance, dietitians who actually go to markets in an ethnic neighborhood can see the types of foods available, evaluate their cost, ask other shoppers and store personnel about what conditions they believe the foods are especially good or bad for, and learn about their preferred preparation. Dietitians will be better able to adapt diabetic diets of persons from that ethnic group to the ethnic foods available, their income levels and tastes, and the culturally perceived appropriateness of such foods for diabetics.

When using PO as part of a formal research study, researchers are required to make certain that the persons under study are aware that research is being done, have been apprised of their rights as research participants, and have voluntarily agreed to participate. The ensuing discussion of PO does not encompass all elements of a formal research study. It is merely intended to demonstrate techniques health care professionals can use to help overcome selective inattention. Nevertheless, it is always a good idea to let people know when and why we are observing them, asking them many questions about their common, everyday activities, and engaging in many of those activities with them.

COMMUNICATION CONSIDERATIONS

If people know you are actively trying to learn more about their culture or their feelings about a situation, and you are interested in them as persons, they are more willing to share information with you and to educate you in their cultural beliefs and practices.

Phase One: Complete Observer. The role of a complete observer is like being a passive spectator who is visible but has no direct interaction with those being observed. The complete observer role is advantageous when we know little, if anything, about a group or the cultural rules for and patterns of behavior governing their interactions in RSS. Table 6-1 lists examples of ways you, as a complete observer, can passively obtain basic background information about multiple dimensions of a groups' cultural beliefs and practices. As you do such observations, write notes or memos to yourself (fieldnotes) of questions your observations raise in your mind, or any inferences you draw from them, or hunches you have about their meaning. At a later time, you can ask key informants about your questions, inferences, and hunches.

Table 6-1

Gathering Basic Information About Cultural Groups as a Complete Observer

- Read scholarly texts, articles, reports, or surveys about the cultural group, especially those that deal with health and illness. Most university and public libraries or government agencies have such works available.

- Watch films, television, videos, and stage plays and read fictional novels that deal with the cultural group. (See Appendix II for some ideas.) Foreign language media is an excellent source of such material.

  - Pay particular attention to the context (who, what, where, when, and why) of facial expressions, mannerisms, gestures, and other nonverbal behaviors; tones of voice; gender, spousal, intergenerational, and family roles and relationships; types of health care and resources available; social and welfare issues of importance; cultural meaning and use of food; and formal and informal political processes (what are the politics of what is happening?).

- Read newspapers and literature published by cultural groups to learn about issues of import to them. Such media are found in ethnic neighborhoods at news and book stores; markets and local grocery stores; public transportation stops; restaurants; schools; churches; health care facilities; post offices and other government agencies; gas stations; and auto repair shops.

- Write to national governments of the cultural group's country of origin or call their local consulates or national embassies for information.

- Health care professionals may also assume a more visible complete observer position similar to being a "fly on the wall" or a loiterer just hanging around. The participant–observer is removed from the center of action but is able to hear and see what is happening. Table 6-2 gives examples of how a complete observer can learn about the cultural and contextual dimensions of provider–client interactions in a primary care clinic.

Table 6-2

Gathering Information about Provider–Client Interactions

- Position yourself so that you can observe interactions between health care professionals and clients in a primary care facility. Do note the following information and activities.

- To refresh your memory about the RSS later on, draw a map of the physical setting, marking where essential elements are located (e.g., doors, windows, waiting area, reception and work areas, laboratories, examination and diagnostic rooms, refreshment machines area, toilets, audiovisual viewing areas, trash receptacles, and equipment and storage areas).

- Note how the placement of objects (e.g., chairs, desks, and equipment) and the location of rooms, doors, and windows shape, interfere with, or promote, effective provider–client interactions and other types of interpersonal interactions.

- Mark down who the participants are in this RSS and what forms of interactions they have. For example:
  - Who talks and who listens?
  - Was eye contact made and who made it?
  - What was the speed of the conversation and tones of voice used by each participant?
  - What gestures did the participants use?
  - How did the participants carry themselves when walking?
  - What was their posture when sitting?
  - What was their posture when talking to each other?
  - What forms of physical contact took place? How did participants react to such contact?
  - What was the effect on clients when the contact with health care professionals was neutral, friendly, or impersonal?
  - Were they standing/sitting close together or far apart?

- Did clients in the waiting area interact with each other?
  - What did they speak about?
  - What was their verbal and nonverbal behavior?

- ■ How was their behavior similar and/or different from their behavior when interacting with health care professionals?

- • What was the form and content of health education provided? Who gave it?

- • Did the health teaching seem clear and understandable?

  - ■ Were questions asked of clients to ascertain their prior understanding of the topic?

  - ■ Were attempts made to confirm that the client understood the information imparted?

Similar types of observations can be carried out in other types of RSSs in client care areas and in community settings. Such observations will generate questions to ask key informants to clarify, confirm, or reject preliminary inferences about contextual factors that affect client interactions. They will also provide basic information to explore during other phases of the PO process. This information can be used to further clarify the effects of culture on communication, and to ascertain the rules for transcultural communication between ourselves and others in a variety of RSS.

COMMUNICATION CONSIDERATION

Developing wide-angle lens observation skills is especially important when health care professionals are in a clinical situation where they know very little, if anything, about the culture of the client with whom they are about to interact.

When acceptable cultural rules for and patterns of communication behavior are unknown, your best course of action is to "follow the client's lead" (Andrews & Boyle, 1997; Villaire, 1994).

Example:

- • If the client does not look you in the eyes when speaking, do not look the client in the eyes. Instead, direct your gaze to wherever the client is looking (at the floor, to the wall over the right shoulder, or to the top of the desk).

- If the client speaks slowly and softly, speak the same way.
- If the client does not firmly grip your hand during a handshake, apply the same type of pressure rather than firmly gripping the client's hand.
- If the client defers to a family member when answering your questions, include that family member directly in the client assessment process.
- If the client moves closer to you while responding to your question or engaging you in conversation, do not back away out of the client's comfort zone.

Following clients' leads will convey that you respect them, that you welcome their participation in the assessment process, and that you are willing to learn from them. When it comes to questions about cultural rules for behavior, there is no better way to become competent in the use of culture than for the client to become the teacher and you the learner.

COMMUNICATION CONSIDERATIONS

Just observing a series of interactions that are occurring over and over again is one of the best and most unobtrusive ways to gain a beginning knowledge about behavior. You can then raise questions to ask the people involved to learn more about the meaning of what you saw.

Phase Two: Observer-as-Participant. Observation and interviewing constitute the majority of the participant–observer's time and may be accomplished in two general ways. Health care professionals continue to observe RSS, but they also include interviewing of key informants to clarify impressions and inferences they have made from their previous observations. (See Tables 6-1 and 6-2). A typical sequence of events for this strategy is given in Table 6-3, using the example of clients from a particular cultural group who seldom look directly at health care professionals (HCPs) during verbal exchanges. You can use the same strategies in different types of transcultural communication situations.

Table 6-3

Data Gathering Using Observation and Interviews

STRATEGY	EXAMPLE
Make additional observations in other RSS to confirm your initial observation.	Members of a cultural group seldom look directly at HCPs during verbal interactions.
Make inferences (best guesses) or hunches regarding the meaning of behavior *and*	"I think it means they are shy with strangers." "It could also be a way to show respect to HCPs."
Jot down questions about the behavior to ask key informants *and*	"Is it due to shyness?" "Is it a way to show respect?" "Is it a form of politeness?" "Does it mean they agree or disagree with HCPs?"
Consult the literature or other sources of data for information about the cultural group.	What have others learned about nonverbal behavior, facial expressions, eye contact, and talking with HCPs?

Interview key informants:
    First, briefly summarize the
    inferences/hunch and
 	
    then
	Ask the questions about the preliminary inferences/hunches you wrote down. "I have noticed that clients from this cultural group do not look at HCPs when they are speaking. Why is this?"

Based on the explanation given, ask more focused questions to get specific information about aspects of the behavior.	"When is it proper to look directly at someone when talking?" "How does age, gender, or position of authority affect whether they look directly at people when talking?"

Table 6-3 (Continued)	
STRATEGY	EXAMPLE
Summarize the answers of each key informant and confirm them to be sure you have accurately understood them.	"Based on what you said, looking directly at someone means *(summarize each meaning obtained)*."
Make inferences about the behavior you believe members of the cultural group expect of you in various RSS, and confirm them with your key informants.	"When I do teaching, I should avert my eyes to *(whatever the acceptable cultural behavior is)*." "When I greet clients who are older than me, I should do *(whatever the acceptable cultural behavior is)*."
Test out the newly formed rules for cultural behavior by making repeated observations in a variety of similar RSS with various types of clients from the same cultural group.	Ask yourself if their behaviors are what you expect based on your newly learned rules for and patterns of cultural behavior.
If the actual behavior is repeatedly inconsistent with expected behavior, note differences and contextualize them. Test them out again by consulting key informants and/or making additional observations.	

It is important to remember that people seldom behave exactly the same, even in seemingly identical or similar RSS. Before concluding that your newly learned cultural rules for communication are incorrect, contextualize them. Were there things different in the environment that could have accounted for the client's unexpected behavior?

Example:

- Had the client waited an exceptionally long period of time to be seen?
- Were others present or not present who normally would or would not have been there?

- Was the interaction in the waiting room rather than in the usual and more private examination room?
- Did the client have an unpleasant encounter with someone while registering or waiting?
- Did you appear angry when you entered the examination room or when you greeted the client?

Any one of the above factors or events could influence clients to respond differently (not follow their usual cultural rules for verbal communication).

A second way to be an observer-as-participant is to begin with interviewing and then follow with observations and participation. This is a good strategy when time is limited, an isolated event is experienced or witnessed that is not likely to recur for a long period of time, and/or when something happens that peaks your curiosity. It is also an ideal strategy when you are simply interested in learning about some aspect of another cultural group. Examples of PO that start with interviewing follow.

Action	Example
You enter an ethnic restaurant, note that it is decorated in a festive manner, and members of the ethnic group seem to be celebrating.	When someone comes to take your order do the following. • Ask what the festivities are about. • Inquire about which foods you should order so that you join in celebration like a native. • At some point, ask to speak to a key informant (e.g., the owner, manager, staff member, or another patron) so you can obtain a more in-depth explanation of the who, what, where, when, and why of the celebration. • Take the opportunity to learn about the different foods on the menu. For example: – When are they typically eaten? – Are they from any particular region of the country or special subcultural group (socioeconomic class, occupation, or gender)?

Action	Example
	– Which foods are considered particularly nutritious and why? – Are they associated with any particular event (e.g., holiday, festival, or family celebration)?

Attend a religious ceremony in an ethnic place of worship. Precede this by reading about the religion.	Do the following:
	• Note the events occurring, who is participating in them, and how they act.
	• Speak with a key informant (clergy, worshiper, or ritual assistant) to learn about different aspects of the worship service and the religion.
	  – What do the various symbols mean (e.g., dress, items used in the ceremony, coverings on altars/other structures, paintings, statues, texts, singing, and music)?
	  – What special religious services may be done during illness?
	  – Which religious symbols are used to protect or restore the health of a group/individual?
	  – When are members of the ethnic group likely to seek religious help or guidance?
	  – Who can provide such assistance?
	  – What are the special religious holidays and observances of the group?

Go to arts and crafts festivals held by different ethnic groups or to open-air markets in ethnic neighborhoods.	Ask key informants (e.g., booth operators, artisans present, festival organizers, or patrons) about some of the following: • What is the history and origin of the festival/market? • What does the art or dance symbolize? • What foods are available? – What do they mean in the context of the festival? (See the restaurant example given earlier).

- If there is a health component to the festival/market, gather information about the products available, when they are used, and how they are to be prepared.
  - Explore the who, what, where, when, and why of alternative healing modalities that may be on display.

Similar types of interviewing can be done in conjunction with weddings, funerals, births, coming-out ceremonies, sports, recreational and leisure time events, family gatherings, ethnic pharmacies, and alternative healers or alternative healing establishments.

COMMUNICATION CONSIDERATIONS

Avail yourself of every opportunity to learn about some facet of a group's culture. When learning about cultural characteristics, explore the history of their origin, their meaning, and their relationship to health, illness, and good fortune. It is through endeavors such as these that you can learn the cultural rules for and patterns of behavior, as well as the types of cultural resources within an ethnic community that can be utilized in client care.

Phase Three: Participant-as-Observer. Because you will already know a great deal about the cultural rules for and patterns of communication behavior, this phase requires less detachment or separation of participant–observers from the events at hand than during phase two. Now, you can refine your knowledge and skills by spending a great deal of time in the participant role. Instead of mainly observing client interactions and interviewing key informants in a primary care setting, you can now consciously use the cultural rules for communication behavior that you learned when interacting with and caring for clients.

The participant-as-observer role is a natural progression on the PO continuum. Communication skills and knowledge gained through the observer-as-participant role in phase two becomes the basis for interaction with clients. There are, however, inherent problems in trying to be a participant-as-observer. Completing the task at hand often assumes primacy. When we are directly giving care, we are often so focused on that task that we forget to be alert to or simply have no time to consciously observe our clients' reactions to us or vice versa. Such involvement in the task at hand severely compromises our ability to step out of our insider's role of care giver and into the role of outsider so we can objectively critique our behavior, as well as that of our clients. Nor do we have the time or freedom to observe events affecting the context in which we are giving care.

Despite the disadvantages inherent in the participant-as-observer role, it is a good way for health care professionals to test their ability to apply newly learned transcultural communication skills and knowledge. Methods of overcoming problems of doing two jobs at once or serving two masters are listed in Table 6-4.

Table 6-4

Critiquing the Participant-as-Observer

- With the permission of the other participants in the RSS, have several of your interactions videotaped. Then critique the videos with key informants.

- With their permission, audiotape your interactions with different types of clients. Critique the tapes with the following questions in mind. You may also want to go over the tapes with a key informant and ask:

  - Am I adapting my teaching and assessment interviews to my clients' characteristics (e.g., level of education, developmental stage, knowledge of conditions, the topic at hand, or concept of privacy)?

  - Did I seek out my clients' knowledge, opinions, beliefs, and/or practices before I began my health teaching or prescribed treatment interventions?

  - Am I picking up verbal and nonverbal cues from my clients that indicate if additional information is needed, the teaching is understood, or the topic is causing distress?

- Have a culturally knowledgeable colleague or someone else observe you as you give care. Discuss their impressions of your ability to apply your transcultural communication skills and knowledge, and your clients' responses.

- As soon as possible after a client interaction is completed, sit down and write out or tape record all that you can remember about it. Reread your notes/listen to the tape and embellish upon your original account. Then critique the interaction.

Phase Four: Complete Participant. This phase of PO is generally not advocated as a way to begin learning about transcultural communication behavior. Being a complete participant means that health care professionals would be full-fledged members of the group under study, interact at all levels with all other participants in the RSS, and function in their role as professionals. Full immersion in carrying out work roles and responsibilities increases our selective inattention and constricts our ability to see the RSS through a wide-angle lens. Our tendency is to focus on the immediate tasks needing to be done rather than on concentrating on everything else that is occurring in the context. It is just too difficult to be fully immersed in one's daily work while simultaneously being detached enough from it to observe things objectively, and to be introspective about our actions, thoughts, and feelings.

The various examples just presented are but a small sample of the variety of ways we can use PO to learn about the rules for and patterns of transcultural communication, as well as lifeways of different cultural groups. A variety of other cultural observation exercises can be found in texts by Hunter and Foley (1976), Pedersen (1988), Scrimshaw and Hurtado (1987), and Singelis (1998).

PARTICIPANT–OBSERVATION INTERVIEWING

Interviewing key informants in conjunction with PO is necessary to fully grasp or understand the cultural insider's point of view, the meaning of what is occurring in the RSS, and to contextualize it. Interviewing also helps to clarify the basis of differences that may exist between the cultural outsiders' and cultural insiders' perspectives on RSS. Interviewing can reveal areas where further cultural knowledge is needed before a cultural outsider can behave in a culturally appropriate manner in RSS.

When health care professionals are first learning about a topic, unstructured interviews along the line of friendly conversation are most helpful. The easiest way to learn about a topic is to get people to tell their stories by asking broad-based, open-ended, **grand-tour questions**: "Tell me what you thought was happening when you first began experiencing your symptoms?" or "What is it like to have to care for your ill mother at home?" "How did this affect your family?" These would be good types of questions to use in phase two of PO when you start out with interviews rather than observations.

When conducting unstructured, interactive interviews, the main role of health care professionals is to actively listen and encourage the speaker to continue. This can be done nonverbally via nods of the head, facial expressions, or other gestures. We can also verbally encourage them to go on speaking: "Please, go on." "How interesting. Tell me more." A good way to end such a broad-based or far-ranging interview is to ask, "Is there anything else you can tell me about (whatever the topic is)?" or "What else should I know about (whatever the topic is)?"

Some interviews during the PO process may be more formal; they have a specific purpose and focus and are conducted at a particular time and place, generally of the cultural insiders' choice. Such interviews usually occur when interviewers (cultural outsiders) know the questions to ask but cannot predict the answers. Questions should be arranged in a logical order, cover the entire topic of interest, and be semi-structured to allow clients to freely describe and explain the situation in their own terms. Examples would be: "Tell me what you do to stay so well." or asking mothers, "Please explain what it means when an infant cries." "What should a mother do when babies cry?" "When is it good for a baby to cry?" For further information on interviewing techniques during PO see Hunter and Foley (1976), Morse and Field (1995), Scrimshaw & Hurtado (1984), and Spradley (1979, 1980).

KEY INFORMANTS

The type of key informant may vary with the RSS and phase of PO. Persons who are actually part of the RSS become key informants when participant–observers ask them to explain, clarify, or interpret what they have seen or experienced. At other times, participant–observers may deliberately seek out individuals who can tell them the meaning of what occurred in RSS even though the key informant was not part of it. For instance, women who have breast fed can describe how to wean an infant even though they are not presently breast feeding. They are experts based on their previous experience.

Certain people make better key informants than others. They are persons who are familiar with the RSS, who are willing to talk about it, and who can discuss what is happening without critiquing it. They accept things as they are and will tell you about it without worrying whether it is what ought to be or what they think you want to hear. Additional information about the selection of key informants and their role in PO can be found in Germain (1993) and Spradley (1979, 1980).

TESTING YOUR KNOWLEDGE

Circle the correct answer.

1. The term that best describes the fact that health care professionals do not consciously observe the details in a situation which are not necessary for them to function is
   a. sensory overload.
   b. explicit awareness.
   c. selective inattention.
   d. introspection.

2. Which of the phrases below best describes the role of health care professionals when they are ordinary participants in everyday situations?
   a. investigative reporters
   b. "fly on the wall"
   c. introspective observers
   d. complete participants

3. The phase of participant–observation in which the health care professional is a spectator is
   a. complete observer.
   b. observer-as-participant.
   c. participant-as-observer.
   d. complete participant.

4. Which phase of participant–observation are health care professionals in when they are testing out the accuracy of the knowledge they have gained of the cultural rules for behavior?
   a. complete observer
   b. observer-as-participant
   c. participant-as-observer
   d. complete participant

5. The best type of interview question to ask during the observer-as-participant phase is
   a. broad-based, grand-tour questions.
   b. close-ended, focused questions.
   c. formal, survey questions.
   d. quick answer, yes-no questions.

6. A good key informant is a person who
   a. is new to the cultural group.
   b. has to be persuaded to talk.
   c. is knowledgeable about the situation.
   d. is objective and critical about the culture.

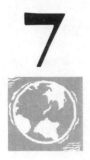

USING BASIC TRANSCULTURAL COMMUNICATION TECHNIQUES

KEY TERMS

- Empathy
- Feedback
- Focusing
- Mirroring
- Rapport
- Reflecting

- Respect
- Restating
- Self-disclosure
- Therapeutic Relationship
- Trust
- Validation

OBJECTIVES

After completing this chapter, you should be able to:

- Recognize the importance of transcultural communication in today's health care system.
- Discuss the goals of therapeutic transcultural communication.
- Identify the three phases of a therapeutic relationship, and describe the goals of each phase.
- Select at least five different approaches that you can use to establish and increase communication in any transcultural interaction.
- Indicate at least five different communication skills that you can use when first meeting a client from another culture.

INTRODUCTION

Earlier chapters have focused primarily on the theory underlying transcultural communication. This chapter will teach you basic transcultural communication techniques that you can use as you work with clients. The importance of clear, sensitive communication during transcultural interactions with clients cannot be overstated. Clear communication is paramount to a harmonious relationship between health care professional and client, especially when the health care professional and the client are from very different cultural backgrounds.

This chapter will teach you the basics of communicating successfully with clients from other cultures. You will learn how to:

1. initiate and build a transcultural, therapeutic relationship

2. develop basic transcultural communication skills

3. perfect specific transcultural communication techniques.

DEVELOPING A TRANSCULTURAL THERAPEUTIC RELATIONSHIP

Because you will be working closely with clients from different cultures throughout your health care career, it is very important to learn how to develop a transcultural therapeutic relationship. At first it may seem difficult to relate in a therapeutic way to people whose cultural beliefs may be very different from your own. Nevertheless, the more you learn about the therapeutic relationship, and the more you practice transcultural communication techniques, the more skilled you will become.

What Is A Therapeutic Relationship?

A **therapeutic relationship** is directed towards helping a client heal, both physically and emotionally. Unlike a social relationship, which is based on friendship and mutual interests, a therapeutic relationship is:

- A professional relationship between a health care professional, (i.e. physician, therapist, or dental hygienist) and a client.

- Focused on helping the client solve problems, and achieve certain well-defined, mutually agreed upon, health-related goals.

- Maintained only as long as the client requires professional help to meet important health-related goals.

The backbone of a therapeutic relationship is *therapeutic communication*. Therapeutic communication is goal-oriented. The goals of *transcultural therapeutic communication* are to help clients from different cultures:

1. explore their life experiences, value and belief systems, and reactions to illness and treatment

2. establish realistic, culturally acceptable, health-related goals

3. take actions that will benefit their physical and mental health, yet still are in keeping with their personal and cultural values.

Phases of a Therapeutic Relationship

Establishing a therapeutic relationship may take days, weeks, or months. As with all relationships, a therapeutic relationship passes through different phases. The four major phases of a therapeutic relationship are (Bolander, 1994; Townsend, 1996)

1. The preinteraction phase

2. The orientation phase

3. The working phase

4. The termination phase.

> *Note:* One major difference between a social and a therapeutic relationship is that in the latter a termination phase is inevitable.

COMMUNICATION CONSIDERATIONS

The successful development of each phase of a therapeutic relationship depends upon the health care professional's communication skills.

Preinteraction Phase. During this phase of the relationship, you will need to learn as much as possible about your client, including reasons for seeking care (see Chapter 10 for detailed information on assessment). To begin your assessment:

- Review the client's medical record and notes.

- Note the client's history of previous health encounters, as well as any procedures that the client has undergone in the past.

- Note the symptoms that brought the client to the clinic or hospital.

- Speak with other health care professionals who may have cared for the client; inquire about the client's cultural background and emotional state, and the client's ability to comprehend his disorder and its treatment.

In addition to learning about your client, you also need to think about your own culturally-based beliefs and values. Honestly examine yourself for any feelings of bias, prejudice, ambivalence, or hostility that you may harbor toward a client of a different race or culture. Of course, uncovering these feelings is only the first step in building a transcultural therapeutic relationship. In addition to facing your feelings of prejudice, you must also be able to put these feelings aside when providing care.

COMMUNICATION CONSIDERATIONS

Remember that any preconceived negative notions that you may have about a client can hinder the development of a therapeutic relationship.

Example: A medical assisting student of Jewish descent had learned as a child that some of her family members had died in the holocaust. While gathering information about a new client, the student discovered that this person was of German descent. The student immediately disliked and distrusted the client. She also incorrectly presumed that the bias she held against the client was also held by the client against her. As a result, the student avoided talking with the client, and failed to gather important client data.

The instructor noticed that the student (who was normally very conscientious) had not completed the client's history. The student finally admitted that she felt uncomfortable with the client because of his German background. The instructor reminded the student that the client was first and foremost an *individual* like herself. The instructor also pointed out that the student was negatively stereotyping the client because of his German background. The student agreed to try and put aside her prejudice and preconceived notions. Once the student made an effort to learn about the client's problems and needs, she began to see him as an individual who was ill and needed her help.

Orientation Phase. During the orientation phase, you need to continue gathering information about your client's history and current problems. This is also the time to: (a) perform a physical, psychosocial, and cultural assessment; (b) formulate client outcomes; and (c) plan interventions. Throughout the orientation phase, it is important to show the client respect, and to establish trust and rapport (see pages 125–127). Also, let clients know that confidential material will be shared only with those individuals who are directly involved in their care.

Working Phase. As soon as you and the client have established a therapeutic relationship, the working phase begins. Now you can begin to:

1. assess the person's concerns, strengths, and weaknesses
2. establish a contract with the client regarding expectations and responsibilities
3. decide on mutually agreed upon goals
4. establish a plan of action that satisfies you and the client
5. set limits
6. discuss the time frame for your relationship. During this phase, continue to establish rapport and build trust, and in doing so, encourage the client to speak openly about feelings, fears, and regrets.

Health needs assessments, plans of action, and evaluations may change as a result of your assessment of the client.

Example: A visiting student from Guatemala was brought into the clinic at the insistence of the American family with whom he was staying. He presented with stomach pains. While the medical assistant was assessing the client, the young man insisted that he wanted to go home without seeing the physician. The medical assistant assessed the client as noncompliant.

However, as the medical assistant asked more questions about health care in Guatemala, she learned that only acute illnesses are considered worthy of treatment. This client did not view his pain as acute and in need of medical attention. Because the client refused treatment due to his cultural background, the medical assistant stopped insisting that he wait for a physician. Instead she had the young man sign a release, instructed him to closely monitor his pain, and advised him to return to the clinic immediately should the pain worsen.

Termination Phase. A therapeutic relationship may be terminated for a variety of reasons: the client may be discharged, the health care professional may change services, or the client's health goals may be met. Regardless of the reason for termination, it should not come as a surprise to the client. Remember that one of the tasks of the orientation phase is to set a time frame for the relationship, and to make certain that the client understands that the relationship will eventually end.

During the termination phase, your major tasks are to:

- Outline the client's strengths and discuss the progress the person has made while in your care.

- Review areas in need of improvement.

- Discuss the client's new goals, and develop a plan of self-care for the client following discharge.

- Discuss any feelings (positive or negative) that the client might have regarding the termination of your relationship.

DEVELOPING TRANSCULTURAL COMMUNICATION SKILLS

Over the past 20 years, thousands of immigrants requiring health care services have arrived in the United States. To work with these culturally diverse groups of clients, health care professionals need strong transcultural communication skills. Health care professionals must know how to communicate clearly with people who speak different languages, and whose cultural backgrounds, values, lifestyles, traditions, and expectations differ (however subtly) from their own.

While you cannot be knowledgeable about every cultural group, it is important to identify those cultural variations that could affect your communication with clients. For example, you should recognize that people from different cultures:

- Differ in their cultural heritage, and thus in their perceptions of illness and treatment.

- Have unique ways of viewing and interacting with health care professionals; for example refugees who have been subjected to imprisonment or torture may view doctors and health care professionals as dangerous authority figures.

- Regard some forms of verbal and nonverbal communication as appropriate, and other forms as not appropriate. Recall from Chapter 3 that some Asians and Native Americans may regard prolonged eye contact as rude.

COMMUNICATION CONSIDERATIONS

The key to successful transcultural communication is to recognize the uniqueness of every culture, every relationship, and every individual—including yourself.

Also, people from different cultures who are ill may have different ways of communicating their fears and needs. Clients may become anxious, resistant, resentful, distrustful, or offended when they feel that health care professionals do not respect their customs, needs, and feelings. Health care professionals can become frustrated and even angry when clients disregard instructions because of a failure to understand or accept the health care professional's verbal and nonverbal communications.

> **Example:** A client who had recently immigrated from Thailand was scheduled for a CT scan. While explaining the procedure to the client, the radiographer often touched the client's head to illustrate that the procedure might cause a severe headache. Suddenly, during this demonstration, the client became withdrawn and anxious. Appearing to be deeply offended, the client refused to listen further to the radiographer, and he also refused the procedure.
>
> The radiographer felt angry, frustrated, and confused. Unfortunately, the radiographer did not realize that in many Asian cultures, the head is a sacred part of the body, and it is considered the carrier of the soul. Thus the radiographer failed to understand that her actions had insulted the client, and devalued his cultural beliefs. Had the radiographer been culturally competent, she would have demonstrated her point with an illustration of a person's head, or pointed to her own head. This simple technique would have helped to establish transcultural communication, and the client would have undergone the procedure.

Establishing Transcultural Communication

Before you can initiate and build a therapeutic relationship, assess clients, or plan and provide their care, you must first establish communication. In other words, your clients must be willing to talk with you, listen to your questions, and give you honest answers. They must trust you enough to tell you about their health history, symptoms, problems, and stresses. They must be willing to listen to your suggestions and follow your instructions. Communicating with clients from different cultures requires sensitivity, knowledge, and skills that can be acquired with study, practice, and experience.

Remember that talking with relative strangers about deeply personal issues is never easy, and it can be particularly difficult for clients who are from different cultural backgrounds than the health care professional. To encourage clients to talk to you about themselves, you must first

1. convey empathy
2. show respect
3. build trust
4. establish rapport
5. listen actively
6. provide appropriate feedback.

Conveying Empathy. **Empathy** involves actively sharing another person's feelings. Empathy can be described as taking on the role of another, and experiencing what that person is experiencing. It is not the same as sympathy, an emotion that involves feeling sorry for someone. Empathy is allowing yourself to enter into another person's emotional experience, while at the same time maintaining objectivity and carrying on your role within the health care delivery system.

COMMUNICATION CONSIDERATIONS

It is important for health care professionals to be empathetic while still maintaining a professional relationship with their clients.

Example: An empathetic medical assistant is able to share the painful emotions of a client who has just received a breast cancer diagnosis, while *simultaneously* helping the person make arrangements for surgery. Unfortunately, because of their own anxieties, some health care professionals are unable to share in the feelings of others, and instead distance themselves from their clients' painful emotions. For example, an anxious medical assistant might efficiently schedule a client's breast surgery, but avoid talking with the client about the disturbing implications of a cancer diagnosis. This distancing on the part of the medical assistant can greatly weaken the bonds of a therapeutic relationship.

Showing Respect. Clients want and need to be treated with respect. **Respect** is more than simply accepting another person; respect is valuing another person and viewing that individual as special. To help clients feel that you respect them, begin by interacting with clients in a formal manner. Members from many Asian and Hispanic cultures respond particularly well to a more formal approach to history taking, assessment, and care. It is also important to show respect for the client's personal space and status. Enabling clients to observe their religious practices and holidays also demonstrates respect.

Older clients, regardless of culture, deserve to be treated respectfully. For instance, although it is a common practice, it is not respectful to address older men or women by their first names, or by nicknames, unless they give you permission to do so. Older people from cultures that hold elders in high esteem may particularly resent being addressed by their first names.

COMMUNICATION CONSIDERATIONS

When you listen to your clients and respect their cultural values and beliefs, you are more likely to gain their trust and cooperation. As a result, clients will be more willing to talk with you about symptoms and problems, and also more motivated to follow your suggestions and instructions.

Building Trust. **Trust** involves having confidence or faith in another person. Trust is a vital component of the therapeutic relationship. Clients who trust you will feel confident that you will watch after their best interests, and that you will also respect their right to privacy and confidentiality. Clients will also feel comfortable discussing their symptoms with you, and even disclosing intimate details of their lives.

However, culture can influence how many personal details a client is willing to share with care providers. For example, Asians typically value a subtle approach to the discussion of problems, and they tend to restrain the expression of strong feelings. Thus Asian clients may find it difficult to speak openly with health care professionals about physical symptoms, or about any mental health problems. Refugees may view you as an authority figure, and thus as a person who cannot be trusted.

COMMUNICATION CONSIDERATIONS

To establish trust with clients, promise no more than you can deliver, keep appointments, and carefully explain procedures and policies—with the help of an interpreter if necessary.

Establishing Rapport. Establishing **rapport** results in gaining your client's trust and acceptance. Rapport is manifested through warmth and friendliness, and the feeling that both people are comfortable with each other. To establish rapport with a client, you might begin by discussing non-health-related topics. For example, you might ask a foreign client where he is from, how long he has lived in the United States, and how he likes living here. If the client appears comfortable with these initial questions, you can then proceed to discuss the person's present symptoms and past medical history.

Listening Actively. Active listening consists of giving verbal and nonverbal clues that communicate that you are interested in the client. When you actively listen to your client, you build trust and show respect. The acronym SOLER is sometimes used to describe those techniques that promote active listening.

S. *Sit* facing the client. This position sends the message that you want to listen to the client, and it tells the person that you are interested in what is being said.

O. *Observe* or maintain an open posture. Sit with your hands in your lap, and your legs uncrossed in a relaxed posture that is non-authoritative and non-threatening. This posture signifies openness, and it will encourage your client to speak freely. Sitting or standing with your hands on your hips, or your arms crossed in front of you is a more authoritative stance which may inhibit the client, or invoke a defensive response.

L. *Lean* toward the client throughout the conversation. This behavior conveys genuine concern and interest. By leaning toward the client, you are showing that you are attentive, and that you sincerely want to understand what the client is trying to tell you.

E. Establish and maintain *eye contact*. Eye contact conveys interest, whereas avoiding eye contact can convey a lack of interest, disrespect, or boredom. Eye contact in the absence of friendliness may give the impression of disapproval. Also, remember that different cultures react to eye contact differently, so you may need to change your communication style accordingly (see Chapter 3).

R. *Relax.* Sit comfortably in your chair and smile in a friendly manner. Communicating a relaxed attitude will help establish a comfortable non-threatening environment in which the client will feel free to speak with you about problems and concerns.

Providing Feedback. Providing a client with **feedback** concerning a modifiable behavior (e.g., disregarding instructions) can help the person change that behavior. Townsend (1996) lists some important points to remember about feedback.

1. Feedback should be used to *describe a behavior,* but not to evaluate (or criticize) the client. In other words, feedback needs to focus on the *behavior* and not on the person. Evaluating or criticizing can put a person on the defensive, which defeats the purpose of feedback.

   Example:
   Description of a behavior: "My nursing assistant mentioned that you didn't want to go to physical therapy. Can you tell me why you didn't feel like going?"

   Evaluation of the person: "Why aren't you cooperating with us? You know that you're supposed to go to physical therapy every day!"

2. Feedback should be *specific* rather than general. Making broad, general statements about the client's behavior is not helpful. Instead, focus on the *details* of a behavior that the client can modify.

   Example:
   Broad Statement: "According to your wife, you are not following your low calorie diet."

   More detailed feedback: "According to your wife, you are still eating a lot of refried beans instead of the black beans we recommended, which are much lower in calories."

3. Feedback should focus on behaviors or situations that the client can *realistically modify.*

   Example:
   Cannot be modified: "You are at risk of high blood pressure because you are a black man."

   Can be modified: "You are at risk of high blood pressure because you are a black man, and you are 30 pounds overweight."

4. Feedback should *provide information* rather than advice. Informative feedback encourages clients to sort out information, and come to a decision on their own.

   Example:
   Providing information: "If you want to lose weight, I can give you a list of the many excellent weight-loss programs that are available.

Be sure to call the programs that you are interested in, and they will give you all of the details."

Advice: "If you really want to lose weight, you should join Weight Watchers."

5. Provide feedback *as soon as possible* following a specific behavior.

Example:

Delayed Feedback: "I noticed last week that you did not bring your daughter into the clinic for her re-evaluation."

Timely Feedback: "I'm calling you because I didn't see your daughter at the clinic this morning. We would like to see her this afternoon or first thing tomorrow. Can you bring your daughter in?"

Using Specific Transcultural Communication Techniques

As you begin your relationship with a client from another culture, plan to use the following basic transcultural communication techniques (Bolander, 1994; Townsend, 1996):

1. When first meeting a new client, *approach slowly* and wait for the client to acknowledge you. Rushing in may exacerbate the fear of the unknown and the unexpected that many clients from other cultures associate with hospitals and health care professionals.

2. *Greet the client respectfully.* Refer to the client by title (Dr., Mr., Mrs.) and last name rather than first name. Make sure that you are pronouncing the client's name correctly. Also, help the client pronounce your name if you notice difficulty in doing so.

3. Provide the client with a *quiet setting* where you will not be disturbed. If the client is confined to bed, draw the curtains completely around the bed to provide privacy. Clients from some cultures may want their families present.

4. Sit a comfortable distance away and lean slightly toward the client. Do not interrupt the client. Avoid changing the subject. Nod occasionally, ask pertinent questions to draw the client out, and—with gestures and facial expressions—indicate that you accept the client's feelings of anxiety, fear, or anger.

5. If your client seems uneasy, pull up a chair and position yourself parallel to and lower than the client. This position helps the patient feel more in control. You may also appear to be more supportive.

6. Allow *sufficient time* for your meeting. Try not to appear rushed or anxious to leave. Avoid fidgeting or looking at the clock. A hurried attitude on your part could offend Hispanic or Asian clients who value politeness, or Native American clients who value an unhurried approach to communication. For example, when assessing a Native American client, do not initially ask questions in a rapid manner. Try a gentler, slower approach. First, identify yourself and then state your name, position, and how long you have worked in the agency or facility. Next, tell the client what you hope to do, and *then* ask questions. Shake hands at the end, not at the beginning of your meeting.

7. *Explain* to clients (especially those who are nervous or fearful) that they can and need to speak freely to you about their symptoms and fears. Emphasize that the information they impart will be shared only with other health professionals for purposes of diagnosis and treatment.

8. *Listen* to what your clients are trying to tell you about their symptoms. Listen with particular care to the words a client uses to describe a symptom. Then use those same terms, rather than medical jargon, when discussing symptoms with that client.

9. Offer the client opportunities to *ask questions*. For example, as you talk with the client, periodically pause to inquire: "Would you like to add something?" or "Do you have any further suggestions?" or "How do you feel about this problem?" This approach should help to increase the exchange of information between you and your client.

   However, culture once again influences whether a client will be quiet during the assessment process or will assertively ask questions. For example, many mainstream white American clients may want to know as much as possible about their condition. Conversely, out of respect, some Asian clients may hesitate to question health care professionals about their diagnoses. However, these Asian clients may still want to know more about their illness. Physicians and other health care professionals need to provide clients with essential information about their diagnoses and health care services, even though some clients may not ask direct questions.

10. Try **self-disclosure** to help establish rapport. For example, if the client is suffering from insomnia, you might mention that sometimes you too are unable to sleep, and you understand how distressing insomnia can be.

COMMUNICATION CONSIDERATIONS

Remember that you should only use self-disclosure to help your client feel more comfortable about providing you with personal information. Once you have established rapport and the client seems comfortable, you should stop talking about yourself, and return the focus of your discussion to your client.

11. Use **mirroring** as another technique to make communication flow more easily. If the client is a Native American who speaks slowly and softly, incorporate that aspect of the client's communication style into your own style. Project calmness in your voice and manner even though you may normally speak rapidly. You might also mirror the person's use of eye contact, increasing or decreasing eye contact as appropriate for that culture.

12. **Focusing** on a single idea or experience mentioned by the client, and then *exploring it further* are two important communication techniques. Delving into experiences, emotions, or ideas in more depth helps those clients who are hesitant to explore certain subjects on their own. While the client may initially find it difficult to talk about a topic, your interest should help the person discuss the matter, and disclose feelings more openly.

Example:

Health care professional (focusing): "Yesterday you mentioned that you were a political prisoner in Tibet before coming to this country. It would be helpful to learn more about your experiences."

Client: "Why should I talk to you about what they did to me and my family? No one believes the torture I've been through."

Health care professional (exploring): "I realize that you have suffered a great deal. I'm very interested in learning more about you and your family, and how you survived, and came to this country. Perhaps we could start by talking about just one incident from your past."

13. **Restating** or *paraphrasing* what the client has said gives the person an opportunity to rethink a statement or idea, and then clarify or change the statement. For example, the client who survived torture might say "I have terrible nightmares every night. Because of these dreams, I can never forget what they did to me." Health care professionals could respond by restating or paraphrasing the client's

words: "Even though you survived, your dreams make you feel like you're still a victim."

14. *Seeking* **validation** from a client ensures that you and your client are talking about the same thing.

Example:

Young black client: "My doctor is really bad!"

White assistant: "Do you mean that your doctor is doing a poor job?"

Young black client. "No! My doctor's great! Black people sometimes say *bad* when they really mean *good. Being bad* is a compliment."

15. **Reflecting** questions or statements back to your clients helps to validate their concerns and fosters confidence. No one wants to be misunderstood, and reflecting shows that you understand and recognize the client's concerns.

Example:

Client: "Should I still use this copper bracelet for my arthritis pain?"

Therapist: (reflecting back the question): "Do you still want to use the copper bracelet?" At this point, the therapist should pause and give the client time to think and respond.

16. Allow *silence* as a communication technique when appropriate (see Chapter 3). Silence gives your client time to reflect and speak. However, clients sometimes use silence to avoid disclosing information about themselves, or as a way to control others. Clients who belong to certain religious groups are sometimes silent because they believe that they are listening to and communicating with God (Davidhizar & Giger, 1994).

Davidhizar and Giger suggest these techniques for responding to a client's silence:

- Avoid interrupting the silence because silence makes you uncomfortable.

- Analyze the meaning of the silence. In the meantime, assess the client's nonverbal communication including the person's posture, amount of eye contact, facial expressions and signs of anxiety.

- Let the client know that you accept the silence. If the client looks thoughtful, you might say: "You seem very quiet. I would like to share your thoughts." If the client looks annoyed or angry, try this approach: "You seem upset. Perhaps we can talk about what is troubling you."

- Provide support if the client acts anxious or fearful. "I can tell that you don't feel like talking right now. That's all right. I'll just sit here with you for a few minutes." This statement may help the client to relax.

- Be silent yourself, and let the client initiate conversation. Sitting quietly with a client may encourage the person to break the silence and communicate verbally with you.

Although there are many reasons for a client's silence, members of some groups (especially Native Americans, Southeast Asians, and individuals from impoverished backgrounds) may not speak because they feel discriminated against or misunderstood. Other clients may feel obligated to keep personal and family concerns private. In this case, reassure the client that you will keep information confidential. Tell your client that you know it is difficult to disclose personal information. To establish rapport and reduce the client's feelings of vulnerability, you might want to disclose some of your own experiences and feelings.

Despite your best efforts, some clients may continue to be guarded and silent. In these cases, you may just have to wait for the person to decide that you are worthy of trust. You may need to defer your questions to a later time.

17. Pay attention to the client's *nonverbal communication,* and it's cultural significance. If you are from a different culture than your client, it may be difficult for you to interpret the meaning of nonverbal communication cues, including:

- quality and tone of voice
- posture
- gestures
- facial expressions
- use of personal space
- use of touch
- frequency of eye contact
- use of communication that is vocal but still nonverbal such as sighing, crying, laughing, moaning, and coughing.

Evaluate the client's verbal communication and nonverbal signals. When verbal and nonverbal signals do not agree (e.g., the client who says he is not nervous but is clearly trembling) ask additional questions to clarify the person's verbal response.

Take care that your normal nonverbal communication does not unintentionally frighten or offend clients from other cultures. As mentioned, mirroring the communication style of your clients is one technique for building trust and reducing the client's anxiety.

COMMUNICATION CONSIDERATIONS

Remember that clients from other cultures may be particularly sensitive to your use of touch and eye contact.

18. *Touch* clients only when you know it is acceptable. As mentioned earlier, the issue of physical contact is indeed touchy. Recall that cultures differ radically as to what kinds of touch are permitted and when. In general, it is more acceptable to touch a child in a comforting manner than an adult. To minimize potential problems, follow these specific guidelines:

   • Many Hispanic clients are accustomed to supportive touch or a gentle embrace. Make a point of shaking hands with Hispanic clients and their families, and of standing or sitting close to the client. It is usually all right to touch an Hispanic client when paying a compliment, because touch is viewed as a gesture of sincerity. When talking to an Hispanic child, praise and smile, while you gently touch the head or hand of the child.

   • Avoid touching a Vietnamese, Cambodian, Hmong, or Thai child on the head during an initial conversation or assessment, as the head has traditionally been considered the site of the soul in these cultures.

   • When touching adolescents, tapping the shoulder or touching the hand is considered appropriate, especially for Filipino, Chinese, Japanese, Southeast Asian, and Hispanic youths. These adolescents are more inclined to exchange hugs amongst themselves, but males may consider obvious signs of emotion as threats to their masculinity.

   • Because the Southeast Asian client may fear bodily intrusion, minimize touching and probing. Carefully explain assessment and treatment techniques before intruding on the client.

19. Remember that the accepted amount of *eye contact* differs between cultures. For example, a lack of eye contact that may indicate emotional problems in a typical American child, may be culturally normal for a child from an Asian household. To help you correctly interpret nonverbal clues, ask the interpreter if the child's behavior is acceptable within the culture, or if the behavior is unique to the child.

Also, recall from Chapter 3 that white Americans generally view eye contact as symbolic of self confidence, honesty, integrity, and attentiveness, while a lack of contact shows disinterest, rudeness, arrogance, and dishonesty. Most Americans and Hispanics are comfortable with eye contact, whereas Asians and Native Americans tend to see eye contact as invasive and a threat to their privacy.

TESTING YOUR KNOWLEDGE

Circle the correct answer.

1. A therapeutic relationship differs from a social relationship. A therapeutic relationship
   a. is a professional relationship between a health care professional and client.
   b. is focused on helping the client solve problems and achieve health-related goals.
   c. ends when the client is discharged, or when the person's health needs have been met.
   d. all of the above.

2. The phase of the therapeutic relationship during which you assess the client, formulate client outcomes, and plan interventions is called the
   a. Preinteraction Phase.
   b. Orientation Phase.
   c. Working Phase.
   d. Learning/Teaching Phase.

3. Feedback should be
   a. general rather than specific.
   b. evaluative rather than descriptive.
   c. informative rather than advising.
   d. delayed rather than immediate.

4. To initially establish communication with clients from other cultures, the health care professional should
   a. greet the client on a first name basis.
   b. lean slightly toward the client throughout the conversation.
   c. hold the client's hand.
   d. convey sympathy to the client.

5. Which one of the following communication skills facilitate transcultural interactions?
   a. mirroring the client's communication style
   b. breaking silences
   c. reassuring the client that "everything is going to be all right"
   d. confronting the client

6. A strategy for communicating nonverbally with clients from other cultures who seem uneasy is to
   a. stand by the client's bedside when speaking.
   b. smile and pat the client's hand.
   c. position yourself parallel to and lower than the patient.
   d. maintain eye contact even when the client tries to look away.

8

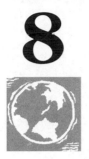

OVERCOMING TRANSCULTURAL COMMUNICATION BARRIERS

KEY TERMS

- Bias
- Dual Ethnocentrism
- Expectations
- Knowledge Deficit
- Language Barrier
- Medical Terminology

- Multiple Realities
- Participant-Observation
- Perceptions
- Perspective
- Stereotype
- Terminology

OBJECTIVES

After completing this chapter, you should be able to:

- Acquire information about the beliefs and values of the specific cultural groups represented in your client population.

- Challenge any cultural biases or ethnocentric attitudes that may interfere with your transcultural communication.

- Explain medical terminology to clients from other cultures in terms that they can understand.

- Identify and overcome differences in how you and your client perceive illness and health care.

- Identify and overcome differences in what you expect, and what the client expects of the Western medical health care system.

INTRODUCTION

Communicating with clients from different cultures may be complicated by (a) the health care professional's lack of knowledge, (b) bias, ethnocentrism, and stereotyping, (c) language differences, (d) differences in terminology, and e) differences in perceptions and expectations (see Chapter 4). The sections that follow contain guidelines for overcoming each of these barriers.

OVERCOMING A KNOWLEDGE DEFICIT

Health care professionals often assess their clients as suffering from a **knowledge deficit**. However, health care professionals themselves may lack important information and knowledge, particularly concerning the cultural groups with whom they work. Health care professionals who are not knowledgeable about a client's cultural values, health beliefs, and patterns of seeking help will not be able to provide the culturally sensitive care that all clients rightfully deserve.

Fortunately there are several ways for health care professionals to learn more about specific cultures. First of all, you can attend classes and seminars that provide valuable information about transcultural communication. Also, there are many textbooks available that describe the history, beliefs, and practices of the major American cultural groups. For example, Chapter 2 in this book discusses the traditional beliefs and values of the mainstream white American, Asian, Hispanic, black, and Native American cultures. However, although textbooks present the facts, they often do not provide the flavor and essence of a culture.

To delve deeper into the heart of a culture, it helps to read novels, short stories, biographies, autobiographies, essays, and poems written by members of a cultural group. Documentaries, films, and television programs that portray different cultures; foreign films; and films that are written, produced, and directed by members of these groups can also broaden your appreciation of America's diverse cultures. (See Appendix II for examples.) In addition, blacks, Hispanics, and Asians all have their own newspapers, magazines, and radio and television stations that present pertinent issues as well as entertainment. The internet is another valuable tool for learning more about different cultural groups. (See Chapter 6 for more details on these methods for gathering information).

In addition to reading, listening to, and viewing information about different cultures, you will also need to involve yourself in a chosen culture as a participant observer. Recall from Chapter 6 that **participant-observation** (PO) is a modified form of an anthropological method for gaining a relatively rapid understanding of different groups, settings, cultural beliefs and practices, and modes of communication. Chapter 6 provides detailed instructions on how to gather information as an (a) complete observer, (b) participant-as-observer, (c) observer-as-participant, and (d) complete participant.

CONTROLLING BIAS, ETHNOCENTRISM, AND STEREOTYPING

Bias, ethnocentrism, and stereotyping are barriers to transcultural communication because they each act to distort our perception of other cultures (Thelan, 1997). In Chapter 4, we define **bias** as the tendency to view one's own cultural values as better than the cultural values of other people. According to Agar (1997) it is impossible for health care professionals to completely overcome their personal biases when caring for clients from different cultures. What health care professionals can do, however, is to bring their biases to consciousness, and then try to control these biases when working with clients (Charonko, 1992).

> **Example:** Many health care professionals educated in the United States are heavily biased toward Western medicine. When caring for a client from a different culture, American health care professionals need to acknowledge the *client's* traditional health care beliefs and permit the client to follow those beliefs, provided they do not interfere with the client's medication and treatment program. If the client's health practices conflict with Western medical practices, the health care professional should explain the problem to the client, and then make adjustments that will be *mutually acceptable* to the client and the health care professional.

Health care professionals must also recognize that "**multiple realities** operate simultaneously in any health care situation" (DeSantis, 1994). In Chapter 4, we introduced the concept of **dual ethnocentrism**, which involves the health care professionals assessing and evaluating the client's cultural beliefs, at the same time that the client is evaluating the professional's beliefs. According to DeSantis, these client encounters involve the interaction of three separate cultures or realities:

1. The **care provider's** professional knowledge, based on an education in Western medicine, as well as personal beliefs and practices;

2. The **client's** view of Western medicine, based on cultural background and beliefs; and

3. The **setting** in which the client and health care professional are interacting—for example, the hospital, clinic, community, or home and family setting. Institutions such as these have their own rules and expectations about those responsibilities and standards of care which affect the relationship between the client and health care professional.

Health care professionals who understand these multiple realities should be able to view clients from diverse cultures in a clearer light. For instance, clients whom health care professionals have labeled as *noncompliant* may simply be adhering to their own cultural beliefs rather than to hospital policy and the health care professional's biomedical beliefs.

COMMUNICATION CONSIDERATIONS

 To acknowledge that clients have the right to their own health care beliefs is a major step toward overcoming personal and professional biases and ethnocentrism.

Overcoming the tendency to **stereotype** people from different cultures is also very important. Catch yourself before you make statements such as "*All* blacks do this…", Mexicans *always* do that…" and "Native Americans *never* understand this…" In addition, gently correct other health care professionals when they make stereotypical statements about clients with different racial/ethnic backgrounds.

Example: Kathy Ballard (medical assistant) is giving her report to Ken Nickols (physician).

Kathy: "Ken, we just admitted Maria Sanchez again. She's a 62-year-old woman with congestive heart failure. She understands a little English, but she only speaks Spanish."

Ken: "So we'll need to find an interpreter to help with her assessment."

Kathy: "Definitely. *(Sighing)* I don't know about you, but I get so tired of people who immigrate to this country and then they don't learn the language—and then we have to find interpreters! It seems like the Mexicans, in particular, never bother to learn English."

Ken: "Well, I haven't worked in this hospital as long as you have Kathy, but my experience has been different. I've met many Mexican clients who speak very good English."

Kathy: "Why don't they all learn to speak English?"

Ken: "Kathy, listen to yourself! Many Mexicans work two jobs in order to support their families here and help out their families in Mexico. They don't have the time or the money or the energy for English lessons. They have more urgent priorities than learning English."

Kathy: "OK, OK, you've made your point. I admit many Mexicans do speak English, and I guess those that don't have their reasons. I'll call for an interpreter. Why don't you go in and meet Ms. Sanchez. She's probably getting anxious."

OVERCOMING LANGUAGE BARRIERS

Of all the hurdles that health care professionals and their clients must clear in order to communicate, **language barriers** are possibly the most difficult. Language barriers can create many frustrating problems.

- Language barriers can make it difficult or impossible to obtain a client's history and assess the client's symptoms.

- Language barriers can interfere with explaining institutional policies and medical procedures.

- Language barriers can severely impede the vital processes of teaching and counseling the client and family.

- Language barriers, as exemplified in the previous section, can create misunderstandings and resentments between health care professionals and clients.

It is so important to learn how to overcome language barriers, that an entire chapter has been devoted to the subject. Chapter 9 will give you clear guidelines for communicating with clients who have limited English proficiency. This chapter also discusses the client's legal right to have an interpreter, as well as the complex role of the medical interpreter.

OVERCOMING TERMINOLOGY DIFFERENCES

In addition to language barriers, communication problems also arise when clients and health care professionals use different terminology. Most clients—regardless of cultural background—find it difficult to discuss their health problems in the precise clinical terms used by health professionals. First of all, clients tend to focus comments on their discomfort ("It hurts to move my shoulder") whereas health care professionals focus on the resulting functional limitations such as "impaired physical mobility related to arthritis."

Furthermore, clients often describe their ailments in highly personalized and often emotional terms such as: *the dreaded pest, my high blood pressure, my heart attack,* or *my sugar diabetes.* These terms contrast to the biomedical terms *influenza, hypertension, acute myocardial infarction,* and *diabetes mellitus.*

Stokes (1977) has compiled this list of medical terms that are used by health care professionals and compared them with equivalent terms used by some black clients (Cherry and Geiger, 1999).

Medical Term	Equivalent Black Term
Pain	Miseries
Syphilis	Bad blood, pox
Anemia	Low blood, tired blood
Vomiting	Throw up
Constipation	Locked bowels
Diarrhea	Running off, grip
Menstruation	Red flag, the curse
Urinate, urine	Pass water, tinkle, peepee

COMMUNICATION CONSIDERATIONS

Listen to the terms that your client uses and use those terms when performing your assessment. Avoid using abbreviations such as TPR and MI without explaining what they mean to the client.

Gibbs and associates (1987) studied clients' ability to understand **medical terminology**. Their results indicated that clients do not make the cultural jump from lay to medical terms easily. Nearly 50% of clients randomly selected in an urban Primary Care Center defined *hypertension* as meaning nervous or upset. One quarter of the sampled clients understood *orally* to mean when to take a medication (for example, on the hour) rather than taking a medication by mouth.

COMMUNICATION CONSIDERATIONS

Clients who have difficulty with English may be particularly confused by medical terms.

Unfortunately, busy health care professionals sometimes fail to explain medical terms to clients. Indeed, it is not unusual for health care professionals to talk "over the heads" of clients as they perform their assessment. This practice can produce feelings of anxiety, fear, and anger—especially in clients who do not speak English fluently. Such negative feelings can result in clients' noncompliance with important treatment recommendations.

Example: Marie Kowalsky, a young mother and a Polish immigrant who had lived in the United States for 4 years, brought her 5-year-old daughter to a pediatric clinic. While Ms. Kowalsky knew some English, it was nevertheless difficult for her to explain her daughter's symptoms to the physician and medical assistant who were examining the child. During the examination, Ms. Kowalsky unsuccessfully tried to communicate her experience of her child's illness, while the health professionals were more concerned with communicating their observations—primarily to each other.

Ms. Kowalsky: (referring to her daughter) "Iwona feels bad. She tells me her head hurts. She cry very hard. She cry all the time. I think her ears hurt."

Physician: "Let's have a look at her ears." He begins to examine the child's ears with an otoscope.

Ms. Kowalsky: "She doesn't come when I call her. I have to make my voice loud."

Physician: (Speaking to the medical assistant) "It's quite red behind this one drum. Looks like otitis media. We caught it early."

Ms. Kowalsky: (very alarmed): "What's wrong with my Iwona? Otitis? What you talking about?"

Medical Assistant: (to Ms. Kowalsky) "Don't worry Ms. Kowalsky. We'll take care of Iwona. She'll be fine."

Physician: (to the medical assistant): "Let's do an audiogram now."

Medical Assistant: (to Ms. Kowalsky) "Please help Iwona get dressed. I'll be back in a minute to take her for an audiogram."

Ms. Kowalsky was confused. She had no idea what an audiogram was, nor did she understand the term "otitis media," but she helped Iwona dress. In a few minutes the medical assistant returned and led Iwona into another room for the audiogram, leaving the mother to anxiously wait alone.

Medical Assistant: (on returning to the room after completing the audiogram) "She (meaning Iwona) had a hard time understanding the directions."

Ms. Kowalsky: "My Iwona is very smart, she understands. She knows more words than me. She can tell me the words."

Medical Assistant: "According to the audiogram, Iwona doesn't hear sounds the same in both ears. She had trouble vocalizing what she does hear."

Ms. Kowalsky: "My Iwona smart, but she does not hear in her ears good. She tells me 'What?' when I tell her come here."

Medical Assistant: "I'll show the results to the doctor."

Ms. Kowalsky didn't realize that she should wait to see the doctor (no one explained this to her) and so she prepared to leave the clinic.

Physician: (stopping the mother in the hallway) "I'm giving you a prescription for Iwona's ears. She'll need to swallow medicine four times a day."

Ms. Kowalsky: (frustrated and bewildered) "Her ears hurt. She have trouble hearing me. How does swallowing pills help her ears?"

Physician: (harried) "Ms. Kowalsky, I wish I had more time to talk with you about Iwona's medication, but I'm really rushed today. When you stop at the pharmacy downstairs, have the pharmacist explain how the medicine works."

Ms. Kowalsky went down to the pharmacy but saw that the waiting room was crowded with clients, all waiting for their prescriptions to be filled. She was exhausted and Iwona was crying.

Ms. Kowalsky: "Come Iwona, we'll go home now. I fix you dinner and we talk to Baba. She'll know what to do for your ears."

Ms. Kowalsky, who did not understand the importance of the antibiotic prescribed by the physician, failed to have the prescription filled. Instead she relied on the folk medicine remedies recommended by her mother.

Two days later, Iwona's ear infection worsened, and Ms. Kowalsky was forced to return to the clinic with her sick child. The medical assistant at the clinic blamed Ms. Kowalsky for not giving Iwona the prescribed medicine. In reality, it was the physician's and medical assistant's responsibility to explain Iwona's illness and its treatment to the mother *in terms she could understand*. For example, the physician could have said:

"Ms. Kowalsky, Iwona has an infection in her ears. It's making her ears hurt and it's making it hard for her to hear. We tested her hearing with a procedure called an audiogram. We found that Iwona didn't hear very well in her right ear.

"We need your help to treat Iwona's infection. This is an antibiotic medication for you to give Iwona by mouth, four times a day. The antibiotic will circulate throughout Iwona's system where it will fight the infection. It's very important that you give Iwona her medicine on time. Also, you must give her all of the pills, even when she starts to feel better.

"Do you have any questions? If you think of a question later call us anytime. We're here to help you."

COMMUNICATION CONSIDERATIONS

To provide optimal care, take the time to explain medical terminology, directions, and procedures to your clients in terms they understand. Encourage clients to ask questions and express feelings and concerns.

OVERCOMING DIFFERENCES IN PERCEPTIONS AND EXPECTATIONS

All communication between the health care professional and client is to some extent *bicultural*, even when health care professional and client are from the same culture. The client's **terminology**, **perspective**, **perceptions**, and **expectations** represent the lay culture whereas the health care professionals' terminology, perspective, and perceptions represent the subculture of health care. When clients and health care professionals are also from different cultures, communication problems are compounded.

Even when your clients understand medical terminology, their perceptions of illness and health care may be different from yours. These differences can lead to serious misunderstandings during the assessment and treatment process—especially when you are working with clients who adhere to traditional cultural values and behaviors.

> **Example:** On a home visit to the Morales family, a home health aide found a pair of sharp scissors under the pillow of 4-month-old Anna, and removed them. The home health aide, who assumed that Mrs. Morales was being careless, emphatically told the mother to put the scissors away before the infant had an injury. Actually, Mrs. Morales was following an ancient Aztec tradition of leaving needles in the form of a cross under a pillow to ward off evil. Some people who adopted this custom used open scissors (that resemble a cross) in place of needles to keep evil away.
>
> The home health aide was surprised when Mrs. Morales began to cry. The home health aide responded that Mrs. Morales was crying because she had realized that the scissors might have injured her child. The home health aide left the home feeling satisfied that she had prevented an injury. Mrs. Morales, who was angry at the aide for not respecting her traditions, immediately replaced the scissors under her child's pillow.

In this situation, the home health aide would have communicated more effectively with the mother had she asked questions rather than simply assuming that Mrs. Morales was being irresponsible. For instance: "Mrs. Morales, is there some reason that you put scissors under your baby's pillow?" After hearing the mother's explanation, the aide might add: "I now realize that the scissors have an important meaning for you. However, we don't want your baby to cut herself. Is there a safer item that we can put under the baby's pillow? If not, is there someplace else that we can put the scissors? Do you feel satisfied with this solution?"

By acknowledging Mrs. Morales' perception of the scissors and their importance, the home health aide could have corrected a potentially hazardous situation without offending and alienating the mother.

Serious misunderstandings also arise when clients *misinterpret* your clinical assessment findings and recommendations. In one case, a medical assistant in an Adolescent Clinic told the mother of a 13-year-old boy: "Your son has a positive culture for strep throat. You'll need to bring in your other children right away for throat cultures."

The mother (who knew nothing about throat cultures or strep throat) interpreted the medical assistant's request to mean that she had

1. neglected her son (who was now ill)

2. had probably neglected her other children

3. must now bring all of her children immediately to the clinic for testing.

Upset and anxious, the mother did not comply with the medical assistant's recommendation.

To avoid this misunderstanding, the medical assistant needed to clarify her recommendations as follows: "Your son has strep throat, which can be a very serious infection if it's not treated quickly. This infection spreads easily from person to person. Your other children have been exposed to the germs. Please bring your children in so that we can culture their throats for strep. If your children have strep, we will treat them right away. Let's culture your throat as well. Do you have any questions?"

Different expectations of the health care professional's role may also lead to conflicts. For example, clients who use traditional and folk systems of care are not used to a biomedical approach to diagnosis and treatment. They may be suspicious of health care professionals who perform systematic assessments prior to giving care, and may respond to questions with silence.

Furthermore, some clients may believe that your assessment questions indicate that you lack the knowledge to help them. This problem often arises when assessing clients who are refugees or recent immigrants and who still adhere to traditional beliefs.

Rural Alaskan Natives and Native Americans who have received health care only during emergencies (including being driven or air-lifted to a hospital) may expect you to rapidly provide care without asking questions, as in an emergency setting. These clients may be reluctant to give a detailed history and to answer questions because they expect a quick assessment.

COMMUNICATION CONSIDERATIONS

To reduce incompatibilities in transcultural communication:

1. *Strive to understand the client's perceptions and expectations of you and the biomedical health care system.*

2. *Take the time to elicit information about the client's health care belief system.*

3. *In simple terms, carefully explain your role in the assessment process and why it is vital that the client answer your questions.*

4. *Welcome questions from your client and answer them as clearly and simply as possible.*

5. *Allow the client's traditional healer to visit the hospital; let the client follow the traditional healing practices provided that they do not interfere with the prescribed treatment regimen.*

6. *If the client's health care practices do conflict with biomedical practices, communicate with your client until you develop a plan of care that is acceptable to you, the client, and the physician.*

TESTING YOUR KNOWLEDGE

Circle the correct answer.

1. The concept that health care professionals assess and evaluate clients' cultural beliefs at the same time that clients evaluate their health care professionals' beliefs is called
   a. cultural blind-spot syndrome.
   b. dual ethnocentrism.
   c. mutual bias.
   d. dual racism.

2. The statement "Jewish people are always very well educated" is an example of
   a. cultural bias.
   b. a cultural stereotype.
   c. ethnocentrism.
   d. reverse racism.

3. To overcome differences in terminology between you and the client, you should
   a. use the correct medical terminology, and carefully explain the meaning of each term to the client.
   b. give the client a list of medical terms and definitions.
   c. listen to the terms your client uses, and then use those terms when communicating with the client instead of medical terms.
   d. attempt to mimic the client's general language style when communicating.

4. In the example of Ms. Kowalsky and her daughter Iwona, the medical assistant and physician failed to communicate with Ms. Kowalsky because they
   a. failed to define medical terms for Ms. Kowalsky in terms she could understand.
   b. failed to explain the audiogram procedure to Ms. Kowalsky.
   c. failed to give Ms. Kowalsky home care instructions for her daughter.
   d. all of the above.

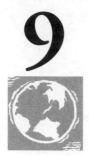

CHAPTER

9

WORKING WITH AND WITHOUT AN INTERPRETER

KEY TERMS

- Communication Barrier
- Equivalent Meaning
- Office for Civil Rights (OCR)
- Professional Medical Interpreter
- Telephone Interpretation Service
- U.S. Department of Health and Human Services (HHS)

OBJECTIVES

After completing this chapter, you should be able to:

- Discuss the role of the medical interpreter, and describe what duties lie within the province of the interpreter's job.
- Differentiate between interpretation and translation.
- List the major provisions of the Code of Ethics for Interpreters in Health Care.
- Identify three vital reasons why medical interpreters are needed in the clinical area, and provide examples of each.
- Discuss a client's legal right to an interpreter if the client does not speak English.

- Describe techniques that will help you to work successfully with a trained medical interpreter.
- Describe techniques that will help you communicate without the aid of a trained interpreter.

INTRODUCTION

Communicating with clients from different cultures is often complicated by language differences. In the preceding sections on communication, we primarily discussed situations in which the client and the health care professional spoke and understood the same language. Health care professionals face a far greater challenge when they try to communicate with clients with limited English proficiency or with no proficiency in English. Unless you learn ways to overcome language barriers, your customary assessment and teaching skills will be seriously hampered, and the client's care may be compromised.

This chapter describes the important role of the medical interpreter, and outlines specific techniques for working with and without a medical interpreter when assessing clients and providing care.

WORKING WITH A MEDICAL INTERPRETER

When the client does not speak English or has limited English proficiency, the best solution is to use a **professional medical interpreter**. To benefit from the services of an interpreter, it is important to understand exactly what an interpreter does, and why a trained interpreter should be used to interpret, rather than family members or other unqualified people.

The Role of the Medical Interpreter

The Code of Federal Regulations defines a qualified interpreter as "an individual who is able to interpret receptively and expressively, using any necessary specialized vocabulary" (Andrea & Renner, 1996). At a meeting of the National Council on Interpretation in Health Care, attendees agreed that the basic role of the medical interpreter is to facilitate communication between people speaking different languages in a health care setting. Ensuring that people can understand each other is the interpreter's job; the content of what is said is the responsibility of client and provider (Roat, 1998).

COMMUNICATION CONSIDERATIONS

Sometimes health care professionals incorrectly ask interpreters to perform duties that are not a part of their role. For example, it is not appropriate to ask an interpreter to explain diagnoses or procedures, or to act as a counselor. Interpreters help with client assessments and interventions only in that they interpret what the provider and client are saying to each other. The interpreter should stay in the background unless a misunderstanding is occurring between client and provider which the interpreter needs to correct.

A medical interpreter plays a different role than a medical translator. Both interpreters and translators take a concept that is expressed in one language and express it in another language. However, an interpreter takes a *spoken* message in one language and renders it in another. A translator takes a *written* message in one language and renders it in another; for example, a translator may translate a client brochure from English to Spanish. Both interpreting and translating are equally accurate, and both relay the denotative (objective) and cognitive (subjective or emotional) meaning of words (Roat, 1998).

Because language reflects a person's reality, experience, culture, and world view, interpreters do not focus on word-to-word equivalence, but rather on the accurate expression of **equivalent meaning**. Thus an experienced interpreter can serve as a *culture broker* and provide a cultural framework for understanding spoken language. That is, an interpreter can convey not only a client's responses to your questions, but also general information about the client's culture—information that will help in assessment and planning. At the same time, a good interpreter will help the client understand the biomedical terms you may need to use, and the basics of the mainstream health care system. Thus, by linking the two cultures, an interpreter can reduce the chances of conflict between health care professionals and clients, and increase trust.

Some interpreters are better trained as culture brokers than others. Moreover, the health care facilities that employ interpreters may limit what interpreters are allowed to do. Also, understand that interpreters may bring their own biases to a situation. As a result, you may not receive full and accurate information, or the interpreter may provide the client with information that you did not intend for the client to receive. Major interpreter biases include: (Putsch, 1985)

- Religious, ethnic, and political biases.

- Socioeconomic biases (e.g., an interpreter from a well-educated or upper-class background may feel inhibited about literally translating those client statements and beliefs that convey folk practices or superstitions).

- Cultural biases (e.g., the interpreter may speak the same language as the client, but may be from a completely different culture).

Because medical interpreting is just emerging as a field, it does not have a universally accepted code of ethics or training requirements. Cynthia E. Roat, an interpreter training coordinator, has written a code of ethics for interpreters in health care that combines codes of ethics from three American health interpretation programs. In order to evaluate your experiences with medical interpreters, it is important to familiarize yourself with this code of ethics, Figure 9-1.

A MEDICAL INTERPRETER CODE OF ETHICS

A medical interpreter is a specially trained professional who has proficient knowledge and skills in two languages and employs that training in a health-related setting in order to make possible communication among parties using different languages.

The skills of a medical interpreter include cultural competency and awareness and respect to all parties involved, as well as mastery of medical and colloquial terminology, which make possible conditions of mutual trust and accurate communication leading to effective provision of medical/health services.

1. **Confidentiality**
   Interpreters must treat all information learned during the interpretation as confidential, divulging nothing without the full approval of the patient and his/her physician.

2. **Accuracy: conveying the content and spirit of what is said**
   Interpreters must transmit the message in a thorough and faithful manner, omitting or adding nothing, giving consideration to linguistic variations in both languages and conveying the tone and spirit of the original message.

   A word-for-word interpretation may not convey the intended idea. The interpreter must determine the relevant concept and say it in language that is readily understandable and culturally appropriate to

(continued)

Figure 9-1. Medical Interpreter Code of Ethics *Reprinted with permission of Cynthia E. Roat, MPH, Interpreter Training Coordinator, The Cross Cultural Health Care Program, PacMed Clinics, Seattle, WA.*

the person being helped. In addition, the interpreter will make every effort to assure that the patient has understood questions, instructions and other information transmitted by the health provider.

3. **Completeness: conveying everything that is said**

   Interpreters must interpret everything that is said by all people in the interaction. If the content to be interpreted might be perceived as offensive, insensitive or otherwise harmful to the dignity and well-being of the patient, the interpreter should advise the provider of this before interpreting.

4. **Conveying cultural frameworks**

   Interpreters shall explain cultural differences or practices to health care providers and patients when appropriate.

5. **Non-judgmental attitude about the content to be interpreted**

   An interpreter's function is to facilitate communication. Interpreters are not responsible for what is said by anyone for whom they are interpreting. Even if the interpreter disagrees with what is said, thinks it is wrong or even immoral, the interpreter must suspend judgment, make no comments, and interpret everything accurately.

6. **Client self-determination**

   The interpreter may be asked by the client for his or her opinion. When this happens, the interpreter needs to provide or restate information that will assist the patient in making his or her own decision. The interpreter should not influence the opinion of patients or clients by telling them what action to take.

7. **Attitude toward clients**

   The interpreter should strive to develop a relationship of trust and respect at all times with the patient by adopting a caring, attentive, yet discreet and impartial attitude toward the patient, toward his or her questions, concerns and needs. The interpreter shall treat each patient equally with dignity and respect regardless of race, color, sex, religion, nationality, political persuasion or life-style choice.

8. **Acceptance of assignments**

   If level of experience or personal sentiments make it difficult to abide by any of the above conditions, the interpreter should decline or withdraw from the assignment.

   (continued)

Figure 9-1. continued

Interpreters should disclose any real or perceived conflict of interest that would affect their objectivity in delivery of their service. For example, interpreters should refrain from providing services to family members or close personal friends except in emergencies. In personal relationships, it is difficult to remain unbiased or non-judgmental.

In emergency situations, interpreters may be asked to do interpretations for which they are not qualified. The interpreter may consent only as long as all parties understand the limitations and no other interpreter is available.

9. Compensation

The fee agreed upon by the agency and the interpreter is the only compensation that the interpreter should accept. Interpreters should not accept additional money, considerations or favors for services reimbursed by the contracting agency. Interpreters should not use the agency's time, facilities, equipment or supplies for private gain or advantage, nor should they use their positions to secure privileges or exemptions.

10. Self-evaluation

Interpreters should represent their certification(s), training and experience accurately and completely.

11. Ethical violations

Interpreters should withdraw immediately from encounters that they perceive to be in violation of the Code of Ethics.

12. Professionalism

Interpreters shall be punctual, prepared and dressed in an appropriate manner. The trained interpreter is a professional who maintains professional behavior at all times while assisting clients and who seeks to further his or her knowledge and skills through continuing studies and training.

Figure 9-1. continued

Reasons For Using A Medical Interpreter

There are three major reasons for using a medical interpreter:

1. legal reasons
2. quality of care reasons
3. financial reasons.

Legal Reasons. Fourteen percent of Americans do not speak English, and they may be legally entitled to the services of a medical interpreter. Federal laws, as enforced by the **U.S. Department of Health and Human Services (HHS) Office for Civil Rights (OCR)**, state that an individual (or class of individuals) *may not be denied an interpreter* when seeking or receiving treatment at a health care facility that is a recipient of federal funds from HHS. According to the Office for Civil Rights:

> The recipient must have bilingual employees or provide interpreters, translators, and other means to ensure the nondiscriminatory provision of services. Such aids must be provided without additional charge to persons needing them in order to benefit equally from any service, program, or activity.

Furthermore, HHS states "No person may be subjected to discrimination on the basis of national origin in health and human services programs because they have a primary language other than English" (Perkins, Simon, Cheng, Olson & Vera, 1998).

In addition to Federal laws mandating the use of interpreters in institutions receiving federal funds, some states also require the use of an interpreter whenever a communication barrier exists. For example, the California Health and Safety Code, Section 1259, requires that licensed acute care hospitals "have a policy in effect and provide, to the extent possible, interpreters whenever a communication barrier exists." The Code defines **communication barriers** as "barriers experienced by persons who are limited in English-speaking or non-English speaking individuals who speak the same primary language and who comprise at least 5% of the population of the geographic area served by the hospital..." (Andrea & Renner, 1996; California Health and Safety Code, 1995).

Unfortunately, while the Federal Government and many states require hospitals to provide interpreters or risk the loss of government funding, there is still a severe shortage of trained medical interpreters within the nation's health care facilities. First of all, it is difficult to enforce those Federal and State laws that require hospitals to hire trained interpreters. Some states are even slashing their budgets for medical interpreters. (Seattle Post-Intelligencier, 1997).

In addition, some clients who speak little or no English probably do not know their legal rights, and are thus unlikely to file complaints with government agencies. In an analysis of the legal needs of indigent immigrants, researchers found that obtaining health care was the third most common legal problem. They also learned that very few immigrants with legal problems were able to obtain legal help (Perkins, Simon, Cheng, Olson & Vera, 1998).

Quality of Care Reasons. Many grave problems involving quality of care can arise from miscommunications between clients and health care professionals due to language barriers. Some of these problems include the following: (Fein, 1997)

- Physicians do not receive an accurate history from their clients, and consequently they misdiagnose clients.

- Clients do not understand their medication and treatment schedules, and thus fail to follow their treatment regimes.

- Clients agree to procedures and even surgeries without fully understanding the consequences and ramifications of treatment.

- Clients are not aware of and thus fail to seek preventative care.

- Clients, their families, and their health care professionals all suffer from severe frustration as they attempt to cross language barriers without the help of a professional interpreter.

COMMUNICATION CONSIDERATIONS

When there is a large immigrant population and not enough skilled interpreters, client care suffers. Poor clients, in particular, are placed at high risk.

When health care professionals are desperate to find someone to interpret for them, they may ask people to interpret who are not qualified. In one Southern California hospital, nursing managers reported that "health care professionals, physicians, students, housekeepers, janitors, clerks, volunteers, clients' friends, and relatives with very little expertise in the language or in medical terminology were relied on to question clients and translate significant medical information" (Rader, 1988). In a large hospital in New York City, an Emergency Department physician reported being forced to use a Vietnamese restaurant owner to translate over the telephone for his Vietnamese client (Fein, 1997).

In a study of three hospitals in San Diego, California, Emergency Department (ED) professionals found that they needed interpreters for 14 languages—Spanish being the most predominate language. The professionals documented that within the ED, 42% of interpreting was done by family members, while 33% of interpreting was done by nonmedical personnel. The family members were often limited in their ability to understand English, while lay personnel were unable to translate medical terminology correctly. This finding validated the ED's need for trained interpreters with backgrounds in medical terminology (Andrea & Renner, 1996).

COMMUNICATION CONSIDERATIONS

If you are not completely fluent in the client's language, it is always best to seek the services of a professional interpreter. Clients may be reluctant to let you know that they do not understand what you are saying. Gross misunderstandings between clients and health care professionals can lead to grave errors in diagnosis and treatment. Use an interpreter when necessary!

Financial Reasons. When interpreters are not available to facilitate communication between non-English speaking clients and professionals, not only does the quality of care decrease, but the *costs* of care increase. Costs can escalate for the following reasons: (Perkins, Simon, Cheng, Olson & Vera, 1998)

- Non-English speaking clients fail to use preventative measures that could prevent costly illnesses and injuries.

- Clients wait to seek medical treatment until their symptoms have worsened, which increases the cost of care.

- Physicians, unable to obtain a full history from the client, tend to rely on expensive and often unnecessary batteries of tests to make their diagnoses.

- Interventions can take 25–50% longer to produce results because non-English speaking clients may not understand or follow the physician's orders (Hagland, 1993).

- Clients miss crucial appointments with their physicians or nurse practitioners, and thus risk suffering unnecessary relapses, which will cost more money to treat.

- Clients may bring malpractice suits or complaints that will be costly and time consuming to address.

COMMUNICATION CONSIDERATIONS

 If your health care facility serves a multicultural population, and does not employ a trained interpreter, remind administrators that interpreters can both increase the quality and reduce the cost of client care.

Guidelines For Working With A Medical Interpreter

If you have never worked with a professional interpreter before, you may initially find the process difficult, as you are relying on another person for your collection of verbal data. To receive the maximum benefit from the interpreter's services with the least amount of frustration, follow these guidelines:

1. Schedule an interpreter to interpret client assessment questions and explain instructions for diagnostic and treatment procedures, consent forms, and any other materials and issues which require clear communication.

2. If possible, request an interpreter of the same gender and similar age as the client. When assessing clients from some cultures, especially Asian cultures, it may be more helpful to work with an interpreter who is considerably older than the client and thus worthy of respect.

3. To make good use of the interpreter's time, decide beforehand on the questions you will ask the client.

4. Try to communicate with the client while you are waiting for the interpreter to arrive. Many interpreters suggest that speaking a few words in the client's language may help the client to relax. Your health care facility may have a phrase chart or picture cards to help you communicate with clients who do not speak English. Even though you may mispronounce words, an attempt on your part to speak the client's language can help to establish rapport and trust.

COMMUNICATION CONSIDERATION

Never ignore clients because they do not speak your language.

5. If possible, meet briefly with the interpreter before you begin your assessment session with the client. Let the interpreter know what you are planning to ask. If the client's language does not contain English equivalents for certain symptoms or disorders, work with the interpreter to develop a new line of questioning.

   For example, the Navajo language does not have an equivalent term for *allergy*. To compensate for the lack of the word *allergy*, you might ask questions to determine whether the client has had any symptoms of an allergy—such as sneezing, rash, dry mouth, or breathing problems—after taking a medicine.

6. You may want to ask the interpreter for the best way to approach delicate issues such as sexuality, impending death, or informed consent. An experienced interpreter will help you find culturally appropriate ways to ask difficult and personal questions.

7. During the session, face the client. Sitting protocols for interpreters differ in different parts of the United States. In some areas, interpreters sit beside and a bit behind the client. Other protocols place the interpreter between the client and health care professional, forming a triangle.

8. Direct your questions to the client and not to the interpreter. Keep appropriate eye contact with the client when you ask questions, and throughout the responses.

9. Remember that even though the client may not speak English, the person may understand some English. Comments not meant for the client's ears should be left until the interview is over and you are alone with the interpreter.

10. Talk about one symptom or problem at a time. Do not ask: "Do you have pain and does it seem to occur when you cough?" Do ask: "Do you have pain?" "Where does it hurt?" "Do you also have a cough?" "Is your cough causing the pain?" Allow the client sufficient time to answer each question.

11. Use short, concise questions and phrases. Avoid idiomatic expressions or colorful expressions that are culture-bound and may confuse the client. Do not say: "Is this problem a real pain in the neck?" or "Do you have your ups and downs?"

12. Look for changes in the client's expression when the interpreter is explaining your questions. Avoid becoming so preoccupied with note taking that you forget to assess the client's tone of voice, body language, and physiologic symptoms such as increased diaphoresis or frequent sighing.

13. If the client's responses to direct questions are very brief, try a more conversational approach: "Some people tell me this (a symptom) happened to them. Have you had this symptom?"

14. If you think the translated answer is too brief after a lengthy and involved client answer, ask the interpreter why the answer was so brief. A short answer may be the appropriate interpretation.

15. If the interpreter feels that a question is inappropriate or might offend the client, wait and discuss the question with the interpreter following the session. Later, the interpreter may find a way to obtain the information you need without offending the client.

16. Be aware that some interpreters may not always follow the ethical guidelines discussed earlier in this chapter. For instance, they may not convey everything that is being said or they may insert their own ideas. Also, an interpreter may be uncomfortable with the topic of questioning. For example, a young female interpreter may find it difficult to ask a young male client about a sexually-transmitted disease.

17. Listen for new ideas that the client introduces. With the interpreter's help, try to expand on those ideas. Do not just go through a list of prepared questions.

18. Following your assessment session, take a few minutes to review the client's answers with the interpreter. If the client seems tired and you have more questions, you and the interpreter may need to schedule a follow-up session.

WORKING WITHOUT A MEDICAL INTERPRETER

While you should always try to work with a medical interpreter, a trained interpreter may not always be available. This section describes (1) how to find someone to temporarily interpret, and (2) what you can do to communicate with your client while you wait for an interpreter to arrive.

Finding Someone To Interpret

When your client speaks little or no English and a trained interpreter is not available, you will need to find someone to interpret for you. Unfortunately, this complex task tends to fall on the shoulders of anyone who is bilingual and who is readily available—this most often being the client's family and friends. While well-meaning, family members and friends are generally not able to interpret precisely and objectively. They may not speak fluent English themselves, and usually do not understand medical terminology.

Moreover, in some situations, complications and confusion can arise when family members try to interpret. For example, asking a school-age male family member to interpret for his grandmother may be inappropriate because he may:

1. be too young to know terms in his native language for certain conditions

2. be embarrassed by words his grandmother uses or the beliefs she voices

3. not interpret everything you and your client say

4. be put in a difficult position from a cultural standpoint, since interpreting gives him the status normally reserved for the adult head of the household.

COMMUNICATION CONSIDERATIONS

Remember to avoid placing a young family member in the emotional position of interpreting devastating news to an older family member. In this situation, make every effort to find a trained interpreter.

In addition, clients may feel too embarrassed to disclose key information in the presence of their relatives, especially if it is of a delicate or sensitive nature. Then too, relatives may attempt to protect their loved one by correcting the client's statements to sound more normal. For example, a relative may not tell the health care professional that the client is reporting hallucinations or hearing voices. Also, older children may tend to answer for the client rather than interpret what the client actually says—resulting in misleading information and an inaccurate assessment.

Unfortunately, without a professional interpreter, you may be forced to rely on a family member to interpret for the client, especially prior to surgery or other procedures, and in the postanesthesia recovery room while the client is regaining consciousness. In emergency situations, you may have little choice but to relay queries through a family member, unless you can find a *bilingual employee* who understands some medical terminology, or your health care facility has access to a **telephone interpretation service**.

For example, some health care facilities have an account with the *AT&T Language Line*. This nationwide, 24-hour service provides interpreters for approximately 140 languages. Although this service does not take the place of a trained interpreter actually present in the health care setting, it does allow clients who do not speak English to communicate their history and symptoms to health care providers—especially in emergencies.

Because telephone interpreters offer an alternative to having a trained interpreter on staff, they are expensive. Indeed, for small clinics, the cost of this type of service may be prohibitive. Furthermore, the quality of the service varies from interpreter to interpreter. Not all telephone interpreters understand medical terminology. Even those interpreters who do understand medical terms are at a disadvantage, because they are not able to assess verbal clues over the telephone. Finally, some older clients may not want to discuss their symptoms and personal problems with a disembodied voice at the other end of a speaker phone (Fein, 1997; Andrea & Renner, 1996).

Guidelines for Working Without an Interpreter

Occasionally you may not have even a family member or a bilingual employee to interpret for you. What should you do to communicate with your client while you wait for an interpreter to arrive? (Delk-Calkins, 1984; Puterbaugh, 1991).

If the client understands a little English, you may be able to gather useful information without an interpreter by following these guidelines:

- Greet the client respectfully. Be polite and formal, especially with older non-English speaking patients, Hispanics, and Asians.

- Try to identify your client's primary language. If you are familiar with any words in this language, use them to show the client that you are trying to communicate. A simple *buenos dias* or *bonjour* may help to reduce the client's anxiety level.

- In some situations, you might try a third language in order to communicate. For example, if you speak French, you may be able to communicate with a Vietnamese client. Because of the French colonial influence in Vietnam, some Vietnamese refugees may be able to speak or read some French. European clients often speak several languages; for example Polish or Russian clients may also speak French or Spanish. If you took Latin in high school, you may even be able use some Latin terms to communicate with clients who speak the Romance languages (French, Italian, and Spanish) which are based on Latin. For example, the word for *pain* in Latin is *dolor*, in Spanish is *dolor*, and in Italian is *dolari*.

- Speak to the client slowly, clearly, and quietly in English, if this is your only option. Do not shout. Unfortunately, there is a tendency to treat people who do not understand English as though they are deaf. Make every effort to not appear frustrated, irritated, or hurried.

- As with an interpreter, talk about one symptom or problem at a time. Use simple sentences and keep your questions short. Use hand movements as necessary to demonstrate what you are asking. Rather than asking: "Where is the pain and is it sharp or does it throb?" Instead, try: "Point out for me the spot where your stomach hurts." "Does it feel like a knife?" "No? Then does it throb?" As you ask these questions, point to your own stomach, or pretend that you are stabbing yourself with a knife.

- Repeat the same question or sentence before restating it in different words.

- Use more literal expressions, and try to avoid using medical terminology. For example, use *bleeding* or *pus* or *liquid* rather than *discharge*.

- Use picture cards or a phrase chart (using phonetic pronunciation) to verify client information.

- Be aware that some clients may answer *yes* to all of your questions in order to avoid appearing ignorant or rude. Actually, the client may have understood very little of what you have tried to say or demonstrate.

While these techniques may temporarily help you to communicate a little with your client, it is nonetheless critical that you find an interpreter as quickly as possible—preferably a trained interpreter. Check with the administrative office for the names of bilingual employees who understand medical terminology. You might also contact a hospital chaplain or rabbi. These spiritual advisors may speak a foreign language or have contacts with individuals who are proficient in other languages.

TESTING YOUR KNOWLEDGE

Circle the correct answer.

1. In an emergency department situation, the most effective way to collect data from a client who has limited English proficiency is to
   a. ask a bilingual coworker to interpret.
   b. question the client via an interpreter.
   c. point to diagrams or pictures.
   d. ask a family member to interpret.

2. A professional interpreter
   a. can act as a culture broker.
   b. can help you understand a client's cultural background.
   c. can interpret for the client better than a close family member.
   d. all of the above.

3. Interpretation differs from translation in which one of the following ways?
   a. Interpretation is more accurate than translation.
   b. Interpretation provides the cognitive meanings of words, while translation does not.
   c. Interpretation takes spoken words from one language and renders them in another language.
   d. Interpretation takes written words from one language and renders them in another language.

4. When working with an interpreter in a health care professional-client-interpreter interaction, you should
   a. focus on the interpreter.
   b. make written notes of the client-interpreter interaction a priority.
   c. maintain eye contact with the client, and address the client when asking questions.
   d. ask the interpreter to explain diagnoses and procedures to the patient.

5. The Medical Interpreter Code of Ethics states that the interpreter
   a. should give a word-by-word interpretation.
   b. should not give a word-by-word interpretation, but should convey the intended idea of the client or professional.
   c. should not convey statements that could be immoral, misleading, or wrong.
   d. should avoid conveying statements that might offend or upset the client.

UNIT TWO
EVALUATION

EVALUATING YOUR
TRANSCULTURAL COMMUNICATION SKILLS

Exercise One: Evaluating How Comfortable You Feel When Communicating With Clients From Other Cultures

Recall that you performed this exercise before you started Unit Two. By now you should have read all of the chapters in the Unit. Also, you probably have had an opportunity to visit at least one ethnic community, and take care of several clients from different cultures. The statements that follow contain assignments that you may have received in the clinical area or community. Using the five levels of comfort, rate how comfortable you *now* feel about performing each assignment. Compare your current levels of comfort with your earlier levels.

- Level 1: I feel very uncomfortable.
- Level 2: I feel rather uncomfortable.
- Level 3: I feel fairly comfortable.
- Level 4: I feel comfortable.
- Level 5: I feel very comfortable.

1. *Assignment:* Go into a market in an ethnic neighborhood and ask the store personnel about the different foods that are available, and how to prepare them.   **1 2 3 4 5**

2. *Assignment:* Go to an ethnic pharmacy and speak with the pharmacist about which over-the-counter drugs the people in the neighborhood tend to purchase.   **1 2 3 4 5**

3. *Assignment:* Visit a cuandero or folk healer and learn about the various healing modalities that he or she uses.   **1 2 3 4 5**

4. *Assignment:* Assess an older Asian female client who is accompanied by many concerned, attentive family members.   **1 2 3 4 5**

5. *Assignment:* Assess an Italian client who is constantly crying and grabbing onto your hand.   **1 2 3 4 5**

6. *Assignment:* Provide home care to a 4-month-old child whose mother has placed open scissors (resembling a cross) under the child's pillow in order to ward off evil spirits.   **1 2 3 4 5**

7. *Assignment:* Give a complete bath to a Vietnamese woman with the husband and older children present throughout the procedure.

1 2 3 4 5

8. *Assignment:* Have a medical interpreter help you collect verbal data from a client who does not speak English. **1 2 3 4 5**

9. *Assignment:* Assess a client who does not speak English without the help of an interpreter. **1 2 3 4 5**

Exercise Two: Evaluating Your Point of View Toward Transcultural Situations

You also performed this exercise earlier in the self-assessment section of this Unit. Select the one answer that best describes your point of view *now* that you have completed the Unit. There is no scoring for these questions.

1. The health care professional when interacting with clients needs to
   a. elicit the client's perspective about being ill.
   b. share food with the client.
   c. adopt the client's customs.
   d. efficiently manage the care of the client.

2. A culturally sensitive health care professional
   a. is knowledgeable about cultural traits.
   b. adheres to institutional regulations.
   c. adapts communication style to be congruent with the client's expectations.
   d. develops expertise in asking questions to gather client data.

3. The attention that should be allotted to communication in transcultural settings is
   a. little or none as few instances are truly cultural exchanges.
   b. fairly significant because more clients are from diverse cultural backgrounds.
   c. only of consequence in some settings.
   d. extremely important and necessary for holistic care.

4. When working with a client in the emergency room who has limited English proficiency, I would
   a. have a close family member interpret for the client.
   b. rely on a telephone language service for pertinent information.
   c. make an effort to find a qualified interpreter.
   d. attempt to communicate with the client using a phrase chart.

5. When interacting with clients I would
   a. encourage them to express their views of illness.
   b. discourage personal beliefs as they have little connection to the health care plan.
   c. elicit information about their family.
   d. insist that they need to comply with their care plan for their own good.

Exercise Three: Reviewing Your *Transcultural Interaction Diary*

1. Have you had an opportunity to interact with members of an ethnic community? _____ Who were the individuals you interacted with?
   _____

   What did you learn about the culture from each of your interactions?
   _____
   _____

2. Have you succeeded in developing a therapeutic relationship with a client from another culture? _____

   What techniques did you use to establish communication with this client?
   _____
   _____

   Are there other techniques that you might have used to establish communication? _____

   Did you use a process recording format to record your interactions?
   _____

   Did you find that format helpful? _____

3. Did you work on overcoming one transcultural communication barrier every week? _____ Which barriers did you focus on?
   _____
   _____

   How successful have you been in identifying and overcoming these barriers? _____

4. Have you had an opportunity to work with an interpreter? _____

What techniques did you use to facilitate your interaction with the client and the interpreter? _____

_____

Are there any other techniques that you plan to try during future client–interpreter sessions?

_____

_____

_____

Exercise Four: Evaluating Your Knowledge of Basic Transcultural Communication Techniques

Write a brief response to these questions, which are drawn from topics discussed in Chapters 6 through 9.

1. All repetitive social situations (RSS) occur in a *context*. What is a context, and why is context forever changing? _____

_____

_____

_____

2. When health care professionals act as participant–observers, they should try to do the following: (give **one example** of each activity, and note if you have participated in this activity)

a. Overcome selective inattention:

_____

b. Use wide-angle lenses:

_____

c. Be both an insider and outsider:

_____

d. Be introspective:

_____

e. Interview people:

_____

f. Keep fieldnotes:

_____

3. When acting as a *complete observer,* the four methods for gathering basic information about cultural groups are:

   a. _____

   b. _____

   c. _____

   d. _____

4. What are the two general methods for being an *observer as participant?* Give examples of each method.

   a. _____

   b. _____

5. What is the difference between a therapeutic relationship and a friendship? _____

6. List three techniques you can use to establish rapport with clients from other cultures.

   a. _____

   b. _____

   c. _____

7. What communication techniques would you use to learn more about a client who is a recent refugee and a victim of torture? _____

   _____

   _____

8. What techniques can you use to respond to a client's silence?

   a. _____

   b. _____

   c. _____

   d. _____

9. For each of the following transcultural barriers, give an example of the barrier and a technique for overcoming it.

   a. *Knowledge deficit:*

      Example _____

      Technique _____

   b. *Bias:*

      Example _____

      Technique _____

   c. *Stereotyping*

      Example _____

      Technique _____

    d. *Terminology differences:*
        Example _____
        Technique _____
    e. *Differences in perceptions and expectations:*
        Example _____
        Technique _____

10. Language barriers can bring a halt to transcultural communication. To overcome language barriers, it is always best to secure the services of a medical interpreter. The difference between translating and interpreting is:

_____

_____

11. What are the three different interpreting styles?
    a. _____
    b. _____
    c. _____

12. If you wanted to assess a client's symptoms, what would you ask the interpreter? _____

_____

_____

13. If an interpreter were not immediately available, what are two means of acquiring client data?
    a. _____
    b. _____

UNIT THREE

USING TRANSCULTURAL COMMUNICATION TO ELICIT ASSESSMENT DATA

UNIT THREE
ASSESSMENT

ASSESSING YOUR ABILITY TO ELICIT ASSESSMENT DATA

Exercise One: Assessing your Personal Objectives

Now that you have studied the basics of transcultural communication in Units One and Two, it is important to set some new personal objectives. What do you want to gain from studying this unit? Check those points in the following list that apply to you. Also, write down any other personal objectives.

My personal objectives are to:

_____ Learn how to perform a cultural assessment.

_____ Overcome the barrier of cultural blind spot syndrome.

_____ Identify my clients' cultural preferences; for instance, what foods they prefer or religious rituals they wish to observe.

_____ Elicit my clients' explanations for their illnesses.

_____ Learn about my clients' patterns of seeking help for their problems.

_____ Feel comfortable when asking a client's family and friends for information.

My other personal objectives for learning how to assess culturally diverse clients are to:

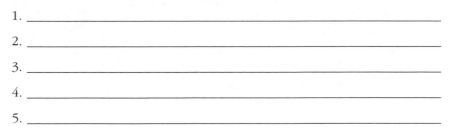

1. _____

2. _____

3. _____

4. _____

5. _____

Exercise 2: Assessing Your Personal Responses to Performing Assessments

More and more of the clients we care for come from cultures other than our own. These clients and their families depend on us to accurately *assess* and *identify health problems and concerns*. How *competent* do you really feel when performing these vital activities? Please take a minute to answer the following questions. You will not need to share these answers with anyone, so try to be honest with yourself.

	Agree	Neutral	Disagree
I should be able to learn how to perform a competent cultural assessment within a few months.	_____	_____	_____
I do not need to culturally assess a client from my own culture.	_____	_____	_____
I need to ask my clients what they believe has caused their illness.	_____	_____	_____
I think that most people do self-care before seeking medical care.	_____	_____	_____

Exercise Three: Using Your *Transcultural Interaction Diary*

1. Before you begin this Unit, please set up a new section in your *Transcultural Interaction Diary*. This section should be devoted to your experiences, thoughts, and feelings when performing cultural assessments.

2. Start working with your diary now, before studying this unit.

3. Before reading Chapter 10, think about the client assessments that you have performed in the past. Were you aware of the vital cultural component that should be a part of all client assessments? Did you ask your clients about their cultural preferences or their views of illness? Did you feel comfortable inquiring about your clients' cultural backgrounds?

4. As you study this Unit, use your diary to record the assessments you perform for people from different cultures. Document the assessments. Write down your thoughts, beliefs, and feelings concerning your assessments. Document how you researched and validated each assessment before implementing care.

5. Continue to keep your diary as you reflect on the information within this Unit. Use the suggested techniques presented in each chapter for improving your ability to assess clients. Note how using a particular assessment technique can help or hinder transcultural communication between you, your client, and your client's family.

10

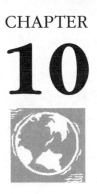

ELICITING ASSESSMENT DATA FROM THE CLIENT, FAMILY, AND INTERPRETERS

KEY TERMS

- Cultural Assessment
- Cultural Blind Spot Syndrome
- Cultural Skill
- Cyclical Pattern of Seeking Help
- Dreyfus Model of Skill Acquisition

- Explanatory Model
- Family Liaison
- Fong's CONFHER Model
- Genogram
- Linear Pattern of Seeking Help

OBJECTIVES

After completing this chapter, you should be able to:

- Identify questions that you might ask clients to determine their cultural backgrounds and preferences.
- Identify and ask questions that will elicit the client's perspective on illness (exploratory model), as well as the family's viewpoints.
- Identify patterns clients use when seeking help.

- Select the important steps you should initially take when eliciting information from the client's family.
- Use various subtle communication approaches when routine elicitation techniques are not effective.
- Culturally assess your clients who are ethnic elders.

INTRODUCTION

Broadly defined, a **cultural** or *culturological* **assessment** is "a systematic appraisal or examination of individuals, groups, and communities as to their cultural beliefs, values, and practices to determine explicit needs and intervention practices within the cultural context of the people being evaluated" (Leininger, 1978). The cultural assessment is vitally important because it helps to ensure that health care professionals will (1) understand and respect each client's cultural beliefs, values, and practices, and (2) take these cultural factors into account when developing a plan of treatment. In support of the cultural assessment, the Joint Commission of Health Care Organizations has concluded that "the impact of the person's culture is an important component of the assessment process..." (Terrance, 1994).

COMMUNICATION CONSIDERATIONS

Remember to do cultural assessments on all clients, including those who are from the same culture as you are. Every client has beliefs and values that are based on culture, and every client is entitled to a cultural assessment. If you fail to conduct a cultural assessment simply because the client is from the same background as you are, you may be falling into the trap of "cultural blind spot syndrome" (Campinha-Bacote, 1995).

Recall from Chapter 4 that **cultural blind spot syndrome** is the belief that "Just because the client looks and behaves much the way you do, you assume that there are no cultural differences or potential barriers to care" (Buchwald, 1994).

For instance, if you are a white health care professional and you are working with a white client, you may incorrectly assume that you do not need to inquire about this client's cultural preferences and beliefs because you are both white. Although white Americans may have many cultural values in common, white Americans also come from a vast array of cultural and religious backgrounds; for example English, Irish, German, French, Amish, and Appalachian backgrounds. To avoid cultural blind spot syndrome, you will need to learn as much about the cultural backgrounds and preferences of your white clients as you learn about your non-white clients.

This chapter will teach you techniques for eliciting information about your clients' (1) cultural backgrounds and preferences, (2) viewpoints concerning illness, and (3) patterns of seeking medical help. This chapter also discusses how to elicit cultural information from the client's family and friends, and how to culturally assess elders from different ethnic backgrounds.

THE ART OF ELICITING INFORMATION

Conducting a successful cultural assessment is an art and a skill that demands knowledge, patience, creativity, and years of practice. **Cultural skill** is the ability to assess clients' cultural beliefs and preferences. In the process of learning how to conduct a detailed cultural assessment, health care professionals seem to pass through five distinct stages before they become experts. The following five levels of experience are based on a modified version of the **Dreyfus Model of Skill Acquisition** that was originally used to study chess players and airline pilots, and later was adapted for health care professionals (Dreyfus & Dreyfus, 1980; Benner, 1984; Campinha-Bacote, 1995).

Level One: Novice

At this level health care professionals have very little cultural skill. They know that they should conduct a cultural assessment, but they do not know how to do so effectively. Novices may feel uncomfortable asking clients what they feel are personal questions. Also, they may fear being viewed by clients as racist. To rise to the next level, novice health care professionals must face and overcome their feelings of discomfort, learn more about the different cultures with whom they have contact, observe how experienced health care professionals conduct a cultural assessment, and find a mentor to help them.

Level Two: Advanced Beginning

Health care professionals at this level are able to conduct a marginally acceptable cultural assessment. By this point, these health care professionals are more culturally conscious than they were as novices. They have attended classes on assessment and are familiar with the different assessment tools. However because they still lack experience, they do everything according to the rules. Advanced beginning health care professionals are afraid to deviate from an assessment tool, and they still lack the skills to think critically and creatively while conducting a cultural assessment.

Level Three: Culturally Competent

At this level health care professionals usually have 2 to 3 years of experience in performing cultural assessments with clients from diverse cultures. Health care professionals who have achieved cultural competency are able to differentiate between important and irrelevant information. They also are more creative in their approach to asking questions, and they no longer need to rely completely on a cultural assessment tool when conducting an interview. However, competent health care professionals are not as confident or as flexible as proficient health care professionals.

Level Four: Proficient

Health care professionals at this level have between 3 and 5 years of experience conducting cultural assessments and are able to evaluate the information they learn from clients in a holistic manner. For example, a novice professional might view client noncompliance as a negative attitude that must be corrected. Proficient health care professionals would recognize that the client is not necessarily being uncooperative, but is simply adhering to cultural beliefs and remedies that differ from those prescribed by the biomedical health care system.

Level Five: Expert

At this level health care professionals are so experienced in performing cultural assessments that they no longer need to rely on specific rules or assessment tools. Because they have interviewed hundreds of clients from different cultures, these health care professionals are able *to intuit* what questions they should ask, and they also know how to seek information in a sensitive manner. Expert health care professionals know what feels right without consciously thinking about what they should ask. To develop their intuitive powers, expert health care professionals must dedicate many years to learning the art of eliciting cultural information from clients, and developing accurate cultural profiles.

ELICITING BASIC CULTURAL INFORMATION

To develop a cultural profile of your client that you can use when planning care, you will need to conduct a thorough cultural assessment. As you ask questions to determine the client's cultural background, values, and current needs and preferences, remember to use the basic transcultural communication techniques that are presented in Chapter 8. Also, to facilitate the assessment process, your health care facility may have a checklist that includes items for client's preferences in diet, personal care, religious beliefs, and so forth. If not, the Cultural Assessment Questionnaire (Figure 10-1) contains sample questions.

The material presented in this figure is partially based on **Fong's CONFHER model**, which provides a systematic framework for organizing your cultural assessment questions and answers. CONFHER stands for the person's Communication style, Orientation, Nutrition, Family relationships, Health beliefs, Education, and Religion (Fong, 1985). In addition to these categories, the Cultural Assessment Questionnaire contains sections of questions concerning occupational and socioeconomic status, personal care, and hospital experiences (Rosenbaum, 1991).

Cultural Assessment Questionnaire

1. Communication
- Do you speak English as your primary language?
- Do you speak another language at home?
- Do you read English? Do you read another language?
- Do you understand common medical terms such as *pain, fever,* and *nausea*?
- Is there a family member to interpret when the hospital (agency) interpreter may not be available?

2. Orientation or Cultural Affiliation
- Where were you born?
- How long have you lived in the United States?
- Were your parents born in the United States?
- How long have your parents lived in the United States?
- Do you or your parents still follow the traditions of your native land (or culture)?

3. Nutrition
- Do you prefer certain foods (vegetarian diet, diet free from pork)?
- Should food be prepared in a certain way (no fried foods)?
- Do you want family members to bring in specific foods?
- Do you abstain from any foods? Do you abstain for religious reasons or for health reasons?

(continued)

Figure 10-1. Cultural Assessment Questionnaire

- How often do you prefer to eat?
- With whom do you usually share your meals?
- What utensils do you prefer to use?
- Are there any foods or drinks that help you to feel better when you are ill?

4. **Religious Affiliation**
   - Do you have religious objects (Bible, amulets) that you want to keep at your bedside?
   - Do you belong to a church group or other religious affiliation?
   - Do you wear clothing with a religious significance (prayer shawl, garment, or cross)?
   - Do you normally pray at certain times during the day?
   - Do you observe the Sabbath or any upcoming religious holidays?
   - Are there any spiritual practices that help you feel better (prayer, meditation, reading scriptures, watching religious programs on television)?
   - Would you like a visit from a representative of your religion?
   - Do you consult a religious healer?
   - Does your religious faith restrict any specific food or drink?
   - Do you fast or refrain from eating certain foods at certain times of the day, week, or month?
   - Are you excused from fasting when ill?

5. **Family Relationships**
   - Who are the members of your immediate or nuclear family?
   - Do you have extended family; in other words, aunts, uncles, cousins, nephews, nieces?
   - Who is the head of household?
   - Who manages the financial matters within your household?
   - Where do you and your family live? In the city or the suburbs?
   - What do you and your family do together for recreation?
   - Do you have family members who will be visiting you in the hospital?
   - How will family members help you during your hospitalization (being present, doing certain things for you)?
   - Who will take over your duties for you at home while you are in the hospital?

6. **Educational Background**
   - What is the last grade or degree that you completed in school?
   - Did you go to school primarily in the United States or elsewhere?
   - Are there any subjects that you have studied outside of school?

(continued)

Figure 10-1. continued

- Are you or your family acquainted with medical terminology?
- Do you learn best from written materials, audiovisual materials, or from a hands-on approach?

7. Occupation and Socioeconomic Status
- What type of work do you do?
- Does anyone else in your family work?
- Do you or your spouse have benefits such as health and dental insurance?
- Do you receive paid sick days, and if so, how many per year?

8. Health Beliefs
- What do you do to stay healthy?
- What do you feel is a healthy diet? Do you try to follow this diet?
- What do you do for exercise?
- Is there anything else that you do to stay healthy?
- Except for this current illness, do you feel that you are reasonably healthy?
- What do you think are the major reasons people become ill?
- Why do you think you have become ill?

9. Hospital Experiences
- Have you ever been hospitalized before?
- When were you hospitalized?
- Where were you hospitalized?
- What was your hospitalization like?
- Is there anything I can do to make this hospitalization easier for you?

10. Personal Care
- Do you prefer to bathe in the morning or the evening?
- Should the nurse follow any special order or routine?
- Do you prefer a family member to assist with your personal care?
- Do you prefer to do as much of your personal care as possible?

Figure 10-1. continued

Sometimes it may be difficult to obtain this valuable personal and cultural data from a client during an initial interview. For example, if the person is admitted with severe chest pain and shortness of breath, you will need to obtain most of the preliminary information from the client's family or friends, and then plan to interview the client later.

Furthermore, you may not be able to conduct an accurate assessment due to language differences. When interviewing a person who does not speak English, remember that it is always best to work with a *trained interpreter* rather than with family members. Unfortunately, many health care facilities do not employ professional interpreters. Chapter 9 describes the techniques that you should use when working with and without an interpreter.

It may also be difficult to obtain complete and accurate cultural information from elderly clients. It may be difficult to interview elderly clients because they may not see or hear well, and some may not own glasses or a hearing aid. Also, ethnic elders may fear your ridicule if they speak honestly about their cultural values and beliefs. To obtain important cultural information from older clients, take care to:

1. Show respect. Always address your elderly clients by their last names unless they give you permission to use first names or nicknames.

2. Use a trained interpreter if the client speaks little English.

3. Provide the client with glasses, hearing aids, or pocket talkers if needed.

4. Interview the client in a quiet setting and provide optimum lighting.

5. Smile and show that you are interested in the client's comfort. For example, provide a warm blanket or a cool beverage.

6. Encourage the client to talk with you about any fears linked to hospitalization or treatment.

7. Note if the client uses hot and cold remedies to treat ailments.

8. If the client sees a non-traditional healer for health problems, ask if the client would like you to call this person and arrange for a visit.

COMMUNICATION CONSIDERATIONS

 When obtaining a medical history from ethnic elders, health practitioners frequently neglect doing a cultural assessment (Evans & Cunningham, 1996).

In addition to these general cultural assessment guidelines, bear in mind the following special precautions:

• Avoid asking a female client from a Far Eastern culture about her reproductive history and related issues in the presence of males. Similarly, an Hispanic woman's modesty may make her hesitant to discuss reproductive or genitourinary concerns with her children present.

• Recognize that in some cultures, including Ethiopian culture, women are socialized to be fragile. You may need to obtain information through her husband or a close male family friend.

- When assessing a Native American client, do not initially ask questions in a rapid manner. Try a gentler, slower approach. First, identify yourself and then state your name, position, and how long you have worked in the agency or facility. Next, tell the client and family what you hope to do, and then ask questions. Shake hands at the end, not the beginning of your meeting.

ELICITING VIEWS OF ILLNESS USING THE EXPLANATORY MODEL

The **explanatory model** (EM), a term used by anthropologists, is the client's explanation for why an illness developed, and conception of how the illness should be treated. The EM interview "is designed to elicit a client's personal, family, social, and cultural beliefs about health, etiology of the illness, onset of symptoms, pathophysiology, course of the illness, and treatment" (Mauksch & Roesler, 1990). The clients who are encouraged to discuss their perceptions of illness and expectations for treatment: (1) experience a greater sense of control and feel more involved in their own care, (2) suffer less from anxiety, and (3) are more likely to accept medical routines and treatment schedules. In sum, clients feel less like powerless pawns that medical personnel push about at random, and more like active members of the health care team.

On the other hand, clients who do not accept the biomedical health care system may hesitate to express health beliefs that are unorthodox or based on folk medicine for fear of ridicule from their health care professional or physician. For this reason, it is very important to ask questions in a sensitive, unhurried way, and to express your respect for the client's viewpoint (Jackson, 1993).

As you assess clients, choose questions that will help you decipher what your clients believe about their current illnesses (Germain, 1992). For example:

- What do you feel caused your illness?

- When and how did your illness begin?

- Why do you think it started when it did?

- How has this illness affected you physically? How has it affected you mentally? Do you feel upset about being ill?

- Has the illness interfered with your job or forced you to change your lifestyle? What course has your illness taken?

- Do you feel ill all of the time? Do you sometimes feel better, and then you have another attack?

- How do you think your illness should be treated?
- What do you think we can do to treat your illness? What are your expectations?
- Do you think that your illness is curable?

COMMUNICATION CONSIDERATIONS

Remember that the concern in your voice is more important than the exact way you word a question.

To further clarify your clients' views, incorporate at least some of the following questions (based on questions asked by health care professionals who triage clients in emergency rooms) into your assessment:

- What do you call this problem you are having? Note: Listen to the client's term and use that term instead of *it* in the following questions.
- When did *it* start and why do you think *it* started when *it* did?
- What problems has *it* brought into your life?
- What problems has *it* caused your family?
- Why do you think that *it* has affected a particular part of your body?
- Why do you think *it* happened to you and not to someone else?
- What have you done to feel better?
- Have you done anything else to feel better?
- Why are you seeking our help to treat *it* now?
- What would you like us to do to help you recover from *it*?
- Are there any other people who are helping you with your problem?

All of these questions may be modified if you are talking to a *parent* or to a *family member* of the client:

- Why did you bring (client's name) to the office, ER, clinic?
- What problem does (client's name) have that concerns you?
- When did (use the term for the illness supplied by the family) start?
- Why do you think *it* started when *it* did?
- Have you done anything to help (client's name) feel better?
- Has anyone else treated your relative?
- What do you hope we can do for your relative?

Some clients may decide to not answer any of your questions because ter-rifying past experiences have made them afraid to talk openly with people in authority. For example, refugee survivors of torture may be reluctant to talk with you about their experiences because they may feel that you will not believe them, or they may be ashamed to talk about what their captors did to them (Chester and Holtan, 1992). In such cases, you might want to try the *indirect approach:*

1. Discuss the problems reported by other clients with similar symp-toms or with the same illness. For example: "Clients who have the same symptoms as you tell me that they also can't sleep. Have you had problems sleeping?"

2. Change a question into a narrative statement. "My clients tell me they sometimes forget to take their medicines. Do you sometimes forget?"

3. Ask if they use a special term to apply to a problem. For example, "Does your language have a term for acute anxiety?" This appeals to your client's cultural beliefs, and seems less direct than asking about a personal problem.

4. Ask the client about his or her general knowledge of a situation rather than specifics. For instance, "I recently read about the harsh treatment of political prisoners in your country. Can you tell me more about this situation?"

5. Use additional questions that focus on family knowledge. For example, "Do any of your family members know what to do to help you with your problem? What has worked for you and your family in the past?"

ELICITING THE CLIENT'S PATTERN OF SEEKING HELP

Recall from our earlier discussions that people from different cultures rely on a variety of methods for seeking medical help. Clients may seek help from the popular sector including:

- Asking advice from family and friends.
- Buying over-the-counter remedies.
- Preparing special diets.
- Participating in exercise programs and/or meditation.

For example, when ill, immigrant clients and clients from refugee groups typically turn first to close family members for help, and then go to the unfa-miliar biomedical care system only as a last resort. People also seek help from such traditional healers as spiritualists, acupuncturists, and curanderos. These traditional healers are esteemed within their culture, and are recognized for their diagnostic and treatment skills.

As noted earlier, clients from different cultures often seek help from more than one source. According to some cultural beliefs, biomedical healers are able to treat the immediate cause of illness, but not the ultimate cause. For this reason, some clients may use the Emergency Department for an acute injury, but visit a spiritualist or acupuncturist for chronic, lingering symptoms.

Clients often use treatment sources in a **linear pattern**—first asking advice from a friend or family member, then going to a biomedical care facility, and then to a traditional healer such as a religious person, a curandero, a spiritualist, or an acupuncturist. Alternatively, clients may follow a **cyclical pattern** of initially seeking biomedical care, then using a traditional healer, and finally returning to the biomedical care system.

Another pattern of care seeking involves the use of *multiple sources of care*. For example, migrant farm workers in California may treat themselves with different available remedies, and wait to seek biomedical health care until they have life-threatening infections or other disabling conditions. Resorting to biomedical care may be late in the client's pattern of health care seeking because (1) workers must depend on their hourly wage to support their families, (2) workers may have limited or no access to affordable health care, and (3) workers usually rely on time-honored alternative treatments that have been transmitted from one generation to another (Jezewski, 1990).

In a study of the use of multiple sources of care, researchers interviewed a group of 203 blacks with hypertension. These individuals initially tried to let their bodies heal through prayer or traditional approaches, such as swallowing a pinch of garlic after eating, or drinking sassafras tea and lemon juice. Next, the individuals evaluated daily activities, sought advice from a family member, and lastly, sought medical assistance (Bailey, 1991).

To assess which methods your clients use for seeking help, ask the following questions (Bushy, 1992):

- Have you done anything to treat the problem?

- What do you do to relieve your discomfort? Does anything you do make you feel better? Is there anything else you do?

- Is there anyone you ask for advice?

- Is there anyone you go to for care besides your medical doctor? Do you seek care from a practitioner, healer, extended family member, or neighbor who is not a medical doctor? Would you like us to contact this person?

- Do you ever go to the drug store or health food store for remedies you can buy over the counter?

- Do you ever try medicines that your family or friends give you?

COMMUNICATION CONSIDERATIONS

 A large portion of clients do self-care, and clients most likely will continue to self-treat while consulting with biomedical health care professionals. Thus, rather than ignoring the fact that your client is self-treating, assess the client's use of self-care, and then consider negotiating a compromise.

Example: A chronically ill 78-year-old man with osteoarthritis was seeking care at an ambulatory care clinic. While taking his history, the medical assistant asked the client why the skin on his wrist was broken and irritated. The client explained that he had been wearing a copper bracelet for his arthritis. He hoped that the bracelet might work, but thus far it had only made his skin sore.

The medical assistant smiled. "I know of other clients who have tried these bracelets. Have you done anything else for your arthritis?" The client replied, "My pain has been so bad that I sprayed my elbow and knee with some lubricant I bought at the drug store. But it hasn't helped much." The medical assistant again asked the client if he had done anything more for the arthritis. The client said that a friend had returned from Mexico with some pills that were supposed to reduce joint swelling, but they were not working either.

Note that by using a non-judgmental approach and by exploring the client's answers in depth, the medical assistant was able to learn a great deal about the client's methods of self-care. Using this information, the medical assistant developed the following client care problem statements:

- Impaired skin integrity related to pressure from copper bracelet

- Risk for infection related to broken skin

- Chronic pain related to chronic disability

Next, the medical assistant in an attempt to negotiate with the client, asked "Are you planning to continue self-treating your joint swelling? If so, are you also willing to take the medication as prescribed?" If the client does decide to use both self-care and biomedical therapies, he may attribute any improvement to his natural remedies.

ELICITING INFORMATION FROM THE CLIENT'S FAMILY AND SUPPORT GROUP

When approached with concern and respect, the client's family can provide you and the physician with vital information. The first steps in working with the family are to (1) survey family members and (2) identify a family liaison.

Surveying the family involves identifying family members and clarifying their relationship to the client. It is important to learn about members of the client's immediate social support network, the client's extended support network, and the client's family history. Surveying is particularly helpful when caring for families in cultural transition (e.g., immigrant families and recently arrived refugees).

In some situations, you may want to develop a **genogram**, which is a tool for recording and visualizing family information. Figure 10-2 provides an example of a genogram. Note that the genogram displays the major illnesses and causes of death among family members, and the age at which each family member died.

COMMUNICATION CONSIDERATIONS

Assure family members that you want to learn about the client's family in order to understand the client's position and role within the family.

Once you become acquainted with the client's family, choose one member to act as a *liaison* to the entire family, both immediate and extended. You will probably select the family member who is the most acculturated to mainstream American values. You can inform the **family liaison** about the client's condition, and ask the liaison to tell other family members. You can also ask that the liaison communicate the ideas and feelings of family members back to you.

To learn about the client's illness from the family's perspective, ask a family member (or the family liaison) the following questions:

- How long have your family members been in this country?

- What are family members doing to help the client deal with pain or other symptoms?

- How has the client's illness affected family relationships? *Note:* In extended families, the client's illness may have disrupted that per-

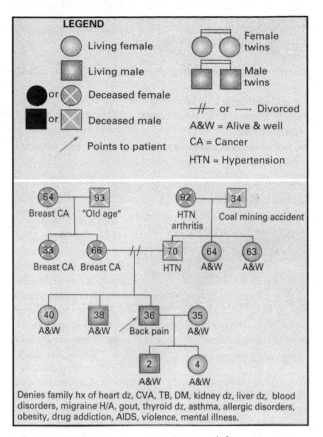

Figure 10-2. A genogram is a tool for organizing and visualizing family information.

son's role (or roles) in the family as primary breadwinner, primary caregiver, or counselor, for example.

- How has the client's illness affected family income? Is the client the primary wage earner? Example: a Cambodian man in his early 20s was hospitalized after being hit by a car. The physical therapist learned that the man had two younger sisters who were attending school, and his elderly father was in poor health. The client was emotionally devastated because he was the primary wage earner in his family. As the client was now hospitalized, he worried that his family would suffer severe socioeconomic stress.

- Do relatives want to be involved in every aspect of decision making that concerns the client?

For instance, in many Hispanic families, the adult children will support each others' decisions regarding care for an aging parent. The son or daughter may request that the health care professional speak with family members first, to protect the client from having to make numerous decisions. This attitude is in contrast to many elderly Greek, East Indian, and Iranian clients who prefer not to discuss any health issues in the presence of their children.

In most cases, family members will be glad to talk to you about their loved one's illness. However, some relatives may be suspicious of an authority figure who asks too many questions—especially immigrant families and refugees who have recently moved to the United States from totalitarian countries. You will need to first gain the trust of families who have experienced life as refugees before they will be willing to share personal information with you.

TESTING YOUR KNOWLEDGE

Circle the correct answer.

1. According to the adaptation of the *Dreyfus Model of Skill Acquisition*
   a. there are three levels through which health care professionals must pass to become experts in cultural assessment.
   b. novice health care professionals rely on their assessment tool and follow the rules.
   c. advanced beginning health care professionals are able to differentiate between important and irrelevant information, and think creatively.
   d. expert health care professionals are able to intuit what questions to ask, and they know what feels right.

2. Health care professionals who are guilty of *cultural blind spot syndrome*
   a. feel that asking clients about their folk beliefs or ethnic practices might appear racist.
   b. believe that it is not necessary to conduct a cultural assessment on a client who is from the same cultural background.
   c. believe that their cultural values are superior to the values fostered by other cultures.
   d. believe that people from other cultures are more spiritual and less materialistic than members of the mainstream white culture.

3. The explanatory model is
   a. the physician's explanation of the etiology of an illness.
   b. a pathophysiologic model.
   c. the client's explanation of illness.
   d. a prioritized flow sheet of interventions.

4. A culturally appropriate approach to assessing a Native American client would include
   a. a firm handshake and direct short answer questions.
   b. an introduction and an indirect line of questioning followed by a handshake.
   c. a rapid interaction.
   d. an interaction focusing on direct eye contact and quick exchange of information.

5. When working with clients who are reluctant to answer questions, you might try an indirect approach by
   a. changing questions into narrative statements.
   b. asking if the client uses a specific term for a problem.
   c. asking the client general questions rather than specific questions.
   d. all of the above.

6. Clients from different cultures who seek help by asking for advice from a friend or family member, then going to a biomedical care facility, and then to a traditional healer are following
   a. a cyclical pattern of care seeking.
   b. a linear pattern of care seeking.
   c. a multi-resource pattern of care seeking.
   d. an alternative pattern of care seeking.

7. Surveying the client's family involves
   a. identifying the client's immediate family.
   b. constructing a genogram.
   c. identifying the client's extended family.
   d. all of the above.

UNIT THREE
EVALUATION

EVALUATING YOUR ABILITY TO ELICIT ASSESSMENT DATA

The following exercises will highlight some of the concepts that were discussed in this Unit. They will also help you identify and evaluate the progress that you have made in your ability to culturally assess clients.

Exercise One: Evaluating Your Personal Objectives

Before you began studying this Unit, you were asked to select and write down your personal objectives for learning about cultural assessments. Please review those objectives now.

1. To what extent have you met each objective that you selected from the list of objectives? _____

_____

2. To what extent have you met the personal objectives that you listed separately? _____

_____

3. What new objectives have you developed since you began reading this Unit? _____

_____

Exercise Two: Evaluating Your Personal Responses to Conducting Cultural Assessments

Now that you have studied this Unit, and have probably had some clinical experience assessing clients, redo Exercise Two from this Unit's self-assessment section. Choose the answer that best describes your point of view *now* that you have finished this Unit, and recorded your experiences in your diary.

	Agree	Neutral	Disagree
I should be able to learn how to perform a competent cultural assessment within a few months.	_____	_____	_____
I do not need to culturally assess a client from my own culture.	_____	_____	_____
I need to ask my clients what they believe has caused their illness.	_____	_____	_____
I think that most people do self-care before seeking medical care.	_____	_____	_____

Exercise Three: Reviewing Your *Transcultural Interaction Diary*

1. What positive experiences (if any) have you had in conducting cultural assessments?

   _____

2. What negative experiences (if any) have you had in conducting cultural assessments?

   _____

3. What difficulties or challenges have you faced as you assessed clients from other cultures?

   _____

   _____

   What do you feel caused those difficulties?

   _____

   _____

   What did you do to overcome those difficulties or challenges?

   _____

   _____

Exercise Four: Evaluating Your Readiness for Conducting Cultural Assessments

Write a brief response to these questions, which are drawn from topics discussed in Chapters 6 through 9.

1. The cultural assessment is vitally important because it helps to ensure that health care professionals:

   a. _____

   b. _____

2. *Cultural blind spot syndrome* is defined as _____

   _____

3. Health care professionals appear to pass through five distinct stages before they become experts at conducting cultural assessments. These stages are:

   a. _____

   b. _____

   c. _____

   d. _____

   e. _____

   f. _____

4. Fong's CONFHER model provides a systemic framework for organizing cultural assessment questions and answers. CONFHER stands for:

   C _____ Example: _____

   O _____ Example: _____

   N _____ Example: _____

   F _____ Example: _____

   H _____ Example: _____

   E _____ Example: _____

   R _____ Example: _____

5. The *Explanatory Model* (EM) is defined as _____

   _____

6. If your assessment indicates that your client is also doing self-care, you should _____

_____

7. A *genogram* is _____

_____

Components of a genogram are: _____

_____

UNIT FOUR

USING TRANSCULTURAL COMMUNICATION SKILLS TO PLAN AND IMPLEMENT CARE

UNIT FOUR
ASSESSMENT

ASSESSING YOUR TRANSCULTURAL COMMUNICATION SKILLS IN PLANNING AND IMPLEMENTING CARE

Exercise One: Assessing How Comfortable You Feel When Planning And Implementing Care for Clients From Diverse Cultures

Planning care, teaching clients, relieving pain, consoling the dying, and assisting grieving relatives and friends are all very important duties. It takes intense study and years of practice to feel truly comfortable when communicating with clients from diverse cultures who need instruction, guidance, and counsel.

This exercise will help you to assess your *current level* of comfort with these transcultural interactions. The following statements contain assignments that you might receive as you work with clients from diverse cultures. Using the following five levels of comfort, rate how you feel about performing each assignment.

- Level 1: I feel very uncomfortable.
- Level 2: I feel rather uncomfortable.
- Level 3: I feel fairly comfortable.
- Level 4: I feel comfortable.
- Level 5: I feel very comfortable.

1. *Assignment:* Talk with a client about his financial and home situation—two factors that can influence your plan of care.

    1 2 3 4 5

2. *Assignment:* Explain to a Japanese client who regularly uses soy sauce and other similar flavorings that he must reduce the sodium in his diet to control his congestive heart failure. **1 2 3 4 5**

3. *Assignment: Negotiate* a biomedical plan of care with a client from a culture that does not totally accept biomedical practices.

    1 2 3 4 5

4. *Assignment:* Witness a client's signing of an *Informed Consent* prior to a major procedure. **1 2 3 4 5**

5. *Assignment:* Develop clear, realistic, and measurable learning objectives for a client who needs to learn about his medications, diet, rest, and activity schedule before going home. **1 2 3 4 5**

6. *Assignment:* Teach a client a procedure such as changing a dressing or self-administration of insulin. **1 2 3 4 5**

7. *Assignment:* Work closely with an interpreter to teach a client with limited English proficiency about his diet and medications.

1 2 3 4 5

8. *Assignment:* Counsel a client with chronic pain who is from a more emotive culture; for example, the Italian culture. **1 2 3 4 5**

9. *Assignment:* Counsel and console a dying client and his family who are observing cultural and religious rituals with which you are unfamiliar. **1 2 3 4 5**

Exercise Two: Assessing Your Point of View Toward Transcultural Situations That Involve Planning, Teaching, Counseling, and Consoling

How do you feel about using transcultural communication techniques to plan care, explain, teach, and counsel clients from diverse cultures? Do you feel that it is very important to consider the client's cultural background when planning and providing care and instruction? Or do you feel that cultural considerations are much less important than other aspects of care? Select the answers that best describe your point of view *now*, before you procede with the chapters in this unit. There is no scoring for these questions.

1. When planning care for clients from diverse cultures, you should
   a. make every effort to preserve the client's cultural practices.
   b. consider the client's cultural practices, but make the biomedical aspects of the client's care plan your major priority.
   c. convince the client that he should follow the biomedical care plan for his own good.
   d. let the client manage his own care as much as possible.

2. A client who refuses to follow a biomedical plan of care
   a. needs to have logical reasons for his refusal to follow the plan.
   b. is being unreasonable and noncompliant.
   c. is observing his legal and constitutional rights.
   d. is recklessly endangering his health, and should be scheduled for a psychiatric consult.

3. When teaching clients from diverse cultures
   a. I try to provide the same information in the same way, regardless of the client's cultural background.
   b. I try to consider the client's special learning needs and limitations that are related to his culture or lack of proficiency in English.
   c. I don't believe that is possible to write measurable learning objectives for clients.
   d. I realize that sometimes it is necessary to negotiate with clients, and must adapt my teaching plan to their cultural views and daily patterns.

4. When caring for clients from diverse cultures who are experiencing pain
   a. I realize that some clients are more stoic in their response to pain, while other clients are more emotive.
   b. it is difficult to evaluate a client's pain when the person responds in a stoic manner, and refuses to acknowledge that the pain exists.
   c. it is difficult to work with clients who scream and cry when in pain.
   d. the client's own description of his or her pain is often inaccurate.

5. When caring for clients from diverse cultures who are dying
   a. I try to accept the client's cultural values and behavior patterns regarding dying and death.
   b. I find it difficult to deal with the dying client's family, when their continuous presence makes it hard for me to provide care.
   c. I don't know what to say when family members express their grief to me following the client's death.
   d. I don't feel that I have the experience to counsel a bereaved family from another culture.

Exercise Three: Using Your *Transcultural Interaction Diary*

1. Before reading the chapters in this Unit, please set up the following four new sections in your diary. Each section should address your feelings,

thoughts, activities, and experiences while: (a) planning care for clients from diverse cultures, (b) developing and implementing a teaching plan, (c) caring for clients in pain, and (d) assisting clients and families as they work their way through the client's death experience.

2. Start recording in your diary *now*, before studying this unit.

3. Before reading Chapter 11, recall and make a note of the times when you have *planned care* for clients from different cultures. Were these experiences positive, neutral, or negative? In each case, how did the client respond to your plan? Did the client totally accept your plan, accept only parts of your plan, or reject your plan? If a client from another culture did reject your plan, how did it make you feel? Concerned? Upset? Angry? Insulted? How did you respond to the client? Did you try to convince him that he was wrong? Or did you try to negotiate and compromise with the client? How did you resolve this situation?

4. Next write down any memorable *teaching experiences*. Have you had an opportunity to develop a formal teaching plan? What types of client teaching have you done? Informal teaching at the bedside? Group presentations? Demonstrations of procedures? Do you feel comfortable teaching clients about their care? If you have had any very positive or negative experiences while teaching, write them down now. Take a few minutes and analyze each teaching experience and your feelings about it.

5. As you study Chapter 11, use your diary to record new experiences as you develop care plans and teaching plans for clients from diverse cultures. Use the transcultural communication techniques suggested in Chapter 11 to help you present your plans to your clients, and to negotiate compromises if necessary. If possible, try to follow your clients' progress even after they leave your health care facility. Try to stay in touch with clients through phone calls, letters, or home visits. Keep a record in your diary of how your clients are utilizing the health care information that you taught them.

6. Before reading Chapter 12, recall and write down your experiences with clients from diverse cultures who were experiencing *pain*. How did these clients respond to their pain? In a stoic manner? In an emotive manner? In each case, how did you evaluate your client's pain? What did you do to relieve the client's pain? In general, were these experiences positive or negative? Take a few minutes and analyze each experience and your feelings.

7. Next write down any experiences that you have had with clients from diverse cultures who were *dying*. Were these experiences positive or negative? Did these clients and their families seem to accept death, or did they refuse to confront death? What cultural and religious practices did the dying client and family observe? Did these practices offer solace and comfort? Were you able to accept these practices and the client's dying wishes? What were you able to do to counsel and console the client and family? Were your actions successful? If so, why?

8. As you study Chapter 12, continue to record your experiences and feelings as you work with clients who are in pain or who are dying. Practice using the transcultural communication techniques presented in this chapter, and then record which techniques were successful for you and which were not. Also, learn all you can about the various ways in which people from different cultures may respond to pain, death, and grief. For example, Asians tend to respond to pain in a stoic manner while Italians are more emotive. Note in your diary if your client's response to pain or critical illness was more in keeping with his culture or with mainstream American culture.

9. As you work with your diary, remember to keep it in a private place. Your diary contains a record of your personal experiences with clients from different cultures. No one should have access to your diary, unless you choose to share it with someone you trust.

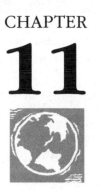
USING TRANSCULTURAL COMMUNICATION TO PLAN CARE, EXPLAIN, AND INSTRUCT

KEY TERMS

- Advance Directive
- Alternative Resources
- Cultural Demands
- Culturally Generated Feelings
- Culture Brokering
- Education by Appropriate Analogy

- Financial Resources
- Informed Consent
- Language Barriers
- Learning Needs
- LEARN Model
- Patient Self-Determination Act (PSDA)

OBJECTIVES

After completing this chapter, you should be able to:

- Use transcultural communication skills when planning care for clients from other cultures.
- Recognize obstacles that you should discuss with clients from other cultures before finalizing their care plans.
- Develop a care plan that is sensitive to the client's cultural needs.

- Appreciate the impact of the Patient Self-Determination Act on the rights of clients to make informed decisions about their own care.

- Identify the client's learning style and use the transcultural teaching method that is most appropriate.

- Teach clients from other cultures how to self-administer medications and assist with or perform prescribed procedures at home.

- Recognize the reasons why clients from other cultures may not comply with your care plan and self-care instructions.

INTRODUCTION

Transcultural communication plays a vital role in all aspects of the health care process. Transcultural communication skills are needed not only for assessing clients from different cultures, but for planning, implementing, and evaluating their care and learning needs.

This chapter, which consists of two parts, spotlights planning and implementation. Part one focuses on using transcultural communication to develop care plans that will be acceptable to clients from diverse cultures. Part two concentrates on implementing care plans. It explores how to use transcultural communication techniques to teach clients about their care and evaluate the results.

TRANSCULTURAL COMMUNICATION IN PLANNING AND IMPLEMENTING CARE

To develop or participate in an acceptable care plan for clients with whom you share cultural values can be quite a challenge. Developing and implementing a care plan for clients from different cultures takes the planning process one giant step further. Not only must the care plan meet the client's needs, but it must also acknowledge and respect the client's beliefs and values. The following sections describe the role of culture in care planning, and provide some specific transcultural communication techniques that will help you develop a plan that your client will accept and follow.

General Considerations

To develop a successful care plan for a client from another culture, you will need to first conduct a thorough cultural assessment (see Chapter 10). It is important to ask clients about their religious beliefs, family relationships, prior hospital experiences, dietary choices, and health beliefs and practices. The more you learn about your client's cultural background and preferences, the more likely it is that your client will find your plan acceptable.

Madleine Leininger has outlined the following three major approaches to planning care for clients from different cultural backgrounds (Jackson, 1993).

1. Make every effort to *preserve* the client's cultural health beliefs and practices that are beneficial. Acupuncture, acupressure, and some herbal medicines are examples of cultural practices that may help clients feel better.

2. *Adapt* or *adjust* the client's cultural beliefs and practices to fit your care plan, provided they are not harmful. The wearing of amulets, certain religious practices, or use of other types of healers in conjunction with biomedical interventions are examples of practices that neither harm nor necessarily help clients. Let your clients know that they are free to observe these cultural and religious practices, but they should also follow their biomedical care plan.

3. Try to *repattern* cultural beliefs and practices that could potentially harm the client's health. For example, Asians traditionally consume foods and flavorings that are high in sodium, such as soy sauce. These food items are dangerous for people with hypertension and heart disease. Although the client may not be willing to completely give up soy sauce, you may be able to persuade the person to use a reduced sodium soy sauce preparation.

Unfortunately, despite your best intentions, care planning may not always proceed smoothly. Clients and their families may not understand or accept biomedical practices or your proposed interventions, and thus fail to follow through on your plan. When your client's health beliefs and practices are at odds with biomedical beliefs and practices, you will need to *negotiate* your care plan through the process of **culture brokering** (See Chapter 9 for more details). Culture brokering is defined as "the act of bridging, linking, or mediating between groups or persons through the process of reducing conflict or producing change." (Chalanda, 1995). A good culture broker (a) respects the values of both cultures and their health care systems, (b) is knowledgeable about both cultures, and c) is able to overcome any existing language barriers, so that everyone clearly understands each other.

Health care professionals who are skilled culture brokers will try to negotiate with the client and family when conflicts arise concerning the care plan. Health care professionals can begin by explaining the biomedical approach to treatment. Next they can inquire about the client's health care beliefs, and ask the client how he feels his condition should be treated. Without trying to change the client's beliefs, health care professionals should encourage the client to think of ways to overcome his objections to the care plan. Whenever possible, it is important to incorporate the client's suggestions into the care plan.

COMMUNICATION CONSIDERATIONS

 The client who is actively involved in making decisions about his health care is far more likely to cooperate with the health care professional's plan of care.

Sometimes, even the most skilled culture broker cannot overcome a client's resistance to a biomedical plan of care. In such a case, it is easy to become frustrated and angry with the client. A client may even be labeled as noncompliant!

Although health professionals may strongly object to a client's decision to reject their plan of care, the fact is that *all clients have the constitutional right to refuse treatment* without giving reasons. Clients are guaranteed this right under the **Patient Self-Determination Act** (PSDA) which was passed by the United States Congress in 1990 and became effective on December 1, 1991.

Since the enactment of the PSDA in 1991, there has been a greater emphasis on obtaining the client's **informed consent** prior to treatment. The consent process ensures that the client has received enough information to make an informed decision about interventions recommended by the physician; e.g., a surgical procedure (Mailhot, 1997). Through the use of **advance directives** (living will or durable power of attorney), the PSDA also guarantees clients the right to make decisions—in advance—about their care should they become mentally incapacitated. For example, some clients may not want to be kept on life support if they have suffered brain damage (Lim, 1997).

In the words of Lawrence P. Ulrich (1994), "The PSDA is a powerful tool in the United States to express society's commitment to personal and cultural diversity and to protect it against violation by those who might think they have a privileged place in society that allows them to dictate to others what is in their best interest."

When a client refuses to follow the plan of care that you and the physician feel is best, what can you do? The first thing you must do is recognize that clients have a right to make health-related decisions that are based on their cultural beliefs and values; after all, it is their life. On the other hand, you do not have to agree with your client's decisions, and you can voice your objections. Nevertheless, you will ultimately need to accept your client's choices. As Charonko points out, "As caregivers our role is to help [clients] live as productively as they can within their own choices. Our role then becomes one of facilitating their efforts to find the resources they will need to meet their goals" (Charonko, 1992).

Specific Techniques

Before beginning to develop your care plan, carefully review all the information about your client that you have gathered during the assessment process. Using your transcultural communication skills, you can then enlarge upon this information as you prepare your care plan. Basic steps in transcultural care planning are as follows:

1. Review the client's *preferences for care*, and then include them in your care plan whenever possible. For example, a client is more likely to follow a prescribed diet if it includes at least some favorite items.

2. Review the client's *cultural preferences*, and make every effort to accommodate those preferences in your plan. A lack of accommodation on your part can lead to resentful resistance by the client and frustration for you. To achieve accommodation, phrase your plan in terms that are consistent with the client's cultural background. You also need to develop a plan that will work within the client's normal cultural environment; for example, within home and work environments.

    Example: Members of some cultural groups believe in the concept that heat and cold are associated with illness. A Pakistani client who had a cold refused to drink the cold juices the nurse assistant offered. It did not make sense to him to treat cold with cold. If a client seems reluctant to take the medications, fluids, or foods that are in his care plan, you might ask the client if he believes in hot or cold notions of illness. The client's decisions regarding what to eat or drink may be based on these beliefs.

3. Address **language barriers** in your care plan. For instance, when you are caring for a client whose native language is not English, include this information in your plan:

Impaired verbal communications related to limited ability to speak or understand the dominant language of the health care delivery system.

On the care plan, you will want to indicate what resources or strengths the person has that will help reduce the language barrier. For instance:

- Client can read simple English phrases.
- Client understands some basic words in English.
- Client can follow short, simple instructions spoken in English.
- Client relies on daughter to interpret. Daughter is available in the evenings for interpretation.

4. Include the client's *family and significant others* in your care plan. Who in the family makes the major decisions? Which family members will be responsible for the client following discharge? What tasks will these family members be expected to perform? Will family members need any special instructions or training?

Also, you will want to investigate how the client's illness has affected family relationships. For example, in extended families the client's illness may have disrupted that person's role (or roles) within the family, such as family head, primary breadwinner, or primary caregiver. Following recovery, the client may need to be reintegrated into his usual family role. If so, you will want to address that process in your care plan.

5. Review the client's *religious beliefs*. In your care plan, note if the client wishes to observe certain rituals or religious dietary requirements. For example, Catholic clients may want to receive daily communion, whereas orthodox Jewish clients will want to observe Jewish dietary laws.

6. Consider the client's *level of knowledge* concerning the disease process and its treatment. If the client is not knowledgeable, you will want to block out ample time to instruct the client about the diagnosis, medications, procedures, and home care.

7. Discuss the **financial resources** that the client must have to comply with a prescribed regimen. If the client appears to have very limited financial means, ask the following:

- Do you receive coupons or vouchers for getting your prescribed medications?

- Have you contacted a local agency for temporary financial assistance?

- Has anyone referred you to an agency that can provide temporary financial assistance?

- Has a nutritionist suggested foods that you can afford? Can you find these items where you shop?

8. Discuss any *other obstacles* that the client faces, such as a lack of child care and/or transportation.

> **Example:** A 14-year-old Alaskan Native American client was discharged from an urban Northwestern hospital with her 3-day-old baby. The medical assistant instructed the young mother to return to the clinic laboratory the next day to have her baby's bilirubin level checked. However, upon further questioning, the medical assistant learned that the mother had been in the city for only 2 weeks, had never ridden on a bus, and had no bus tokens or money for a taxi. The medical assistant had the mother go to Social Services where she received a bus pass.

COMMUNICATION CONSIDERATIONS

 Caution: When questioning a client about available resources, be careful not to simply assume that the client will have problems coping because of youth or poverty.

On the other hand, a 26-year-old mother of four children in a large city was instructed to bring her daughter to the public health department for a dental check-up. Although the mother had already spent her state Aid to Families with Dependent Children grant money, she was resourceful. The mother walked to a social service agency to get bus tokens, which allowed her to keep her daughter's dental appointment.

9. Once you have identified obstacles, look for **alternative resources** available in the client's family and community, and help your client use those resources. For example, you might ask the client, "Do you have a relative who lives near by who can watch your children for a couple of hours while you come to the clinic for treatment?"

10. Be aware of any **cultural demands** that the client faces at home that may compete with important health care needs. When doing discharge planning, ask the client what activities a typical day includes and what role(s) the client plays in the family.

   Example: A visiting nurse assistant was surprised to find her 68-year-old Salvadoran client standing over a stove cooking. The client had recently been discharged following surgery to correct an intestinal obstruction. As the care plan did not state that the woman cared for her three grandchildren while her daughter worked, the nurse assistant had expected to find the client resting. The nurse assistant reported her findings to the home health supervisor who rewrote the care plan, and made arrangements for social services to provide a chore person who could come to the house every day while the client recuperated.

11. Identify any **culturally generated feelings** (e.g., feelings of guilt or shame) that may undermine a client's willingness to follow a health care plan.

   Example: A white middle-class registered dietician (RD) informed a 70-year-old Hispanic male with adult-onset diabetes that he needed to eat a prescribed diet that included more vegetables and less tortillas and beans. During a follow-up appointment, the RD discovered that the client was not following the diet. Careful questioning by the RD revealed that (1) the client lived with his son and daughter-in-law, who did all the food preparation; (2) the daughter-in-law had no idea that the client was to follow a therapeutic diet; and (3) the client was ashamed to admit he needed to diet, especially because it would be more costly for the family to provide.

   In reviewing her notes on Hispanic culture, the RD noted that studies by Albert in 1986 indicated that Hispanics are more interpersonally oriented than whites, and that Hispanic behavior is more frequently related to feelings of shame than white behavior. Recognizing these cultural differences, the RD involved the son and daughter-in-law in the plan of care. She also wrote out suggestions for buying and preparing the prescribed foods at low cost. During the next followup, the RD was relieved to find that the entire family was enjoying meals that included more vegetables and other healthful foods.

12. Respect culturally influenced practices and patterns of behavior that are related to *gender*. For example, female clients from Hispanic or Arabic cultures may feel very uncomfortable in the presence of male health care professionals. In such cases, you might note in your care plan: "Have a female assistant accompany male health care professionals."

13. Above all, recognize your client's concerns, and address them in your care plan.

COMMUNICATION CONSIDERATIONS

Clients may view their conditions differently from health care professionals and they may have different concerns. Some clients perceive the social and psychologic ramifications of their disorders as more important than the medical ramifications that concern health care professionals.

Example: A pharmacist in the Arthritis Clinic of an urban medical center spent a great deal of time discussing possible medication reactions with her clients. However, her elderly clients were primarily worried about how they would care for themselves if they lost their mobility. Because the pharmacist failed to address the client's concerns, they often left the clinic feeling that their real needs had been ignored.

COMMUNICATION CONSIDERATIONS

Communication between health care professional and client must be a two-way process. Although you need to discuss your concerns with clients, it is equally important to listen to their concerns and plan care accordingly.

USING TRANSCULTURAL COMMUNICATION TO EXPLAIN AND INSTRUCT

Transcultural communication provides health care professionals with a powerful tool for implementing their care plans. By using transcultural communication techniques, health care professionals can provide clients from diverse cultures with the vital information they must have to act as partners in their care.

Teaching the client about the care plan can be done on an impromptu basis. For example, while administering medications to a client, you can explain the benefits the person will receive from the prescribed drugs. You can instruct a client in what to expect during a special procedure. While serving a client a special diet, you can discuss which foods are permitted on the diet, which are not permitted, and why.

Client teaching may also be conducted in a more formal manner by using and implementing a written teaching plan. Although providing client education has always been an important health care responsibility, the scope of client education programs were primarily developed by white health care professionals to meet the needs of white clients, or they were modified to meet the needs of ethnic clients by including a token amount of cultural information (Tripp-Reimer & Afifi, 1989). Only within the last decade have health care professionals really tried to address the learning needs of clients from diverse cultures.

The following sections contain basic transcultural teaching principles and special techniques that you can use when instructing ethnic clients.

General Considerations

To successfully instruct clients from diverse cultures, the first thing you must do is establish rapport with your clients by using the transcultural communication techniques described throughout this book. You can use these techniques to do impromptu teaching and to develop planned client teaching programs.

To develop a planned learning/teaching program you will need to (1) assess the client's learning needs; (2) develop a teaching plan; (3) implement your teaching plan; and (4) evaluate your client's progress, making adjustments to your teaching plan as necessary. The sections that follow describe these important steps.

Assess Client's Learning Needs. Before you can proceed to teach, you must first identify your client's **learning needs**. For instance, does the client know anything about the biomedical health care system and how it works? What does the client already know about the disorder? Does the person want to learn more about this illness? Does the client need specific information about a surgery or procedure before signing an Informed Consent Form? Do you need to discuss the benefits of a special diet, or warn the person about possible side effects from medications? Do you need to demonstrate the procedure that the person or significant others will have to perform after discharge?

Note that clients from different ethnic groups may differ in their learning needs. For example, Chinese American clients may want you to explain the cause of illness. Jewish clients may want to know about the actions and side effects of their medications in detail.

Next you need to consider the person's *readiness to learn*. Does the person seem motivated to learn? Does the client want to understand how medications and biomedical treatments will help? On the other hand, is the person too exhausted or in too much pain to concentrate on your explanations? Is the client too anxious to remember your instructions?

COMMUNICATION CONSIDERATION

Before beginning your teaching sessions, make certain that your client is rested and free of pain. If the client appears frightened or anxious, talk with the person about worries and concerns before attempting to teach.

Finally, does the client have any *limitations* that could interfere with learning? For instance, does the client have limited English proficiency? Does the person have limited financial resources and thus is unable to purchase foods for a special diet or buy medications, and thus sees no reason to remember your instructions? Will the client be burdened with work and family responsibilities following discharge, and thus have limited time to follow your schedule for rest and exercise?

COMMUNICATION CONSIDERATIONS

Try to work out ways to resolve the client's limitations before starting to teach. For clients with limited English proficiency, arrange for an interpreter to be present during your teaching sessions. Have a social worker meet with clients who have serious financial problems. Ask for the family's help when clients feel too burdened with responsibilities to follow your instructions and take care of their health.

Develop a Teaching Plan. The next step is to develop a teaching plan. Your teaching plan should be a carefully organized, written presentation that specifies what you want your client to learn, and how you plan to present the information. For instance, you may want your client to learn about how to purchase and prepare the foods on a special diet. Or you may want to prepare for discharge by teaching the client how to change dressings at home. Remember to invite the client's family members to your teaching sessions. Your teaching program will be most successful if the client's family understands how important it is for the client to follow the prescribed treatment regimen.

Your method of teaching should be based on the client's *preferred learning style,* which in turn, may be grounded in the person's cultural background. Many clients prefer to learn with written materials prepared in a language that they can read and understand with ease. Clients from cultures that are characterized by a strong oral tradition may prefer educational films presented in their language. They may also appreciate a group setting where members of the group talk about their experiences, and act as peer educators (Tripp-Reimer & Afifi, 1989). Performing demonstrations and asking for return demonstrations is the best way to teach procedures. **Education by appropriate analogy** provides another method for presenting information.

According to Nichter & Nichter, (1996), education by analogy is "not a new method of education but rather a use of the familiar to explain the new." They further explain that:

> ...a good analogy is like a plow which can prepare a population's field of associations for planting a new idea. If the field of associations is not adequately plowed to accommodate new ideas, it is difficult for such ideas to take root. Equal effort needs to be put into preparing the field, improving the plow, and perfecting the spread of seed.

Here is an analogical message that was developed to teach families in the Philippines birth control by using an intra-uterine device (IUD).

> The IUD is like a fence which the farmer places around his fields to prevent animals from entering and destroying the garden. Placed inside a woman, an IUD prevents her from getting pregnant by preventing the seed from taking root in the uterus.

During the planning period, you will also want to develop some *learning objectives* for your clients. Learning objectives should be clear and realistic. You should also be able to measure your client's progress. The following are examples of learning objectives for Mr. Gonzales, a 65-year-old Hispanic male, who has just been diagnosed with congestive heart failure.

- *Objective 1:* By the end of the first learning session, Mr. Gonzales will be able to explain why it is important for him to eat low-sodium foods and drink low sodium beverages.

- *Objective 2:* By the end of the second learning session, Mr. Gonzales will be able to list the foods, seasonings, beverages, and over-the counter medications that are not allowed on his low-sodium diet.

- *Objective 3:* By the end of the third learning session, Mr. Gonzales will be able to list foods, seasonings, and beverages that are low in sodium. He and his wife will have identified markets where they purchase low-sodium items.

- *Objective 4:* Before being discharged, Mr. Gonzales and his wife will have met with the dietitian, who will assist them in modifying favorite recipes by substituting low-sodium ingredients and seasonings.

- *Objective 5:* During the first home visit, Mr. Gonzales and his wife will have been able to show the health care professional the low-sodium items they have purchased and are now using for meal preparation.

COMMUNICATION CONSIDERATIONS

For learning to take place, the client must believe in your proposed learning objectives as much as you do. For the greatest success, the client needs to be personally involved in the planning stage of your educational program.

Implement and Evaluate the Teaching Plan. Once you have completed your teaching plan and obtained your client's cooperation, you can put your plan into action. You will need to schedule learning sessions with your client and family. If the client has difficulty with English, have an interpreter present during your sessions. It also helps to invite *resource people* to assist you with your teaching. For example, the dietitian can talk with clients about special diets, a physical therapist can teach clients how to do active range-of-motion exercises, and a pharmacist can explain the side effects of medications.

Once the client goes home, it is very important to follow up your teaching with telephone calls, home visits, letters, or return clinic visits. If you are not able to perform follow-up duties yourself, refer the person to the appropriate individuals who can continue to supervise the client's health education. For long-term follow-up, health care facilities sometimes send health education questionnaires to clients.

The final step in the teaching/learning process is to *evaluate* the extent to which the client has met the learning objectives, and has sustained a change in behavior. Changing behaviors takes time, and change is often impeded by occasional setbacks. Food habits in particular are very difficult to change.

When clients experience setbacks, it is important to reassess the client and then evaluate your teaching plan, update it, and implement it again. Because learning is a life-long endeavor, it may take clients many months or even years to make permanent changes in their health-related behaviors.

To summarize, the **LEARN model** (Figure 11-1) developed by Berlin & Fowkes (1993) emphasizes the major steps that are involved in teaching clients from diverse cultures about their health, illnesses, medications, and treatments.

LEARN Model

1. **L**isten and ask questions to assess the client's term for illness as well as what the client believes is causing the illness.

2. **E**xplain (using simple terms) what the client needs to understand about his or her illness. Also explain the reasons for your interventions.

3. **A**cknowledge that the client's views may differ from your own. You probably adhere to the biomedical model of care whereas the client may believe in the traditional model. Take care not to devalue the client's views.

4. **R**ecommend what you would like your client to do. For example, practice drawing insulin or practice changing a dressing.

5. **N**egotiate with the client and adapt your recommendations to the client's views and daily patterns. Have the client assume some control over aspects of the therapeutic plan.

Figure 11-1. LEARN Model. Adapted from Berlin & Folkes (1993).

Specific Techniques

Learning about prescribed medications, new procedures, self-care activities, and important life style changes within the busy and sometimes impersonal medical environment can be confusing and upsetting for any client. But such illness-related experiences are more confusing, stressful, and even frightening when the client is from another culture. The best way to eliminate your client's confusion and fear of the new and unknown is to use transcultural communication techniques. Specific techniques for teaching clients from other cultures include the following:

1. Treat clients as individuals first, while remembering that each client is a member of a cultural group.

2. Follow the general principles of transcultural communication and instruction that were discussed in the preceding sections.

3. Establish rapport with your client. Clients are more likely to learn from you if they like and trust you.

4. Use the client's primary language if possible, but have an interpreter present during your teaching sessions when necessary.

5. Before beginning your explanations and instructions, discuss the client's cultural perspective on illness and therapy. By acknowledging the client's cultural attitudes, you will be able to provide information that the client will understand and accept. As a result, the client will be more willing to make health care choices that you both consider beneficial.

6. When giving instructions, avoid shouting at the client. Instead speak softly and clearly. Your tone of voice should be soothing and convey your intent to help.

7. Reduce the noise level in the room so that the client can concentrate on what you are saying. Recognize that the sound of alarms and monitors can disturb clients, especially those who do not understand the purpose of sophisticated medical equipment.

8. Try to avoid rushing. You can increase the client's level of comfort and readiness to receive and provide information if you can convey that you have time to listen. Remember that communication can be potent therapy.

9. Use simple sentences and ask questions that are brief and to the point. Do not say, "Did you take all of your medicines today or did you miss some?" Rather, "Which medications did you take today?"

10. Repeat instructions, restating them in different words. For example, "Swallow one of these pills every hour until they are all gone.
(continued)

Swallow a pill at 7:00AM, 8:00AM, 9:00AM, and so on until you have swallowed all of the pills."

11. Use more literal expressions—*swallow* rather than *take*; *bleeding* or *pus* or *liquid* rather than *discharge*. Avoid idioms such as *better than nothing* or *start from scratch*.

12. Whenever possible, explain the reason for the client's symptoms prior to discussing a medication, intervention, or procedure. For example, when treating a client with congestive heart failure, try saying:

> Right now your heart isn't able to pump out enough blood to give your body the oxygen and nutrition it needs. This is why you feel so tired. You also have fluid in your lungs, which is making it hard for you to breathe. We're going to give you a daily dose of a medicine called digitalis. Digitalis will help your heart pump better, which will help your blood circulate better. We're also going to give you a water pill. This water pill, or diuretic, will get rid of the extra fluid in your lungs so that you can breathe easier.

13. Take into account the client's explanation of why the illness developed and how it might be treated (see discussion of the explanatory model in Chapter 10). For example:

> I see in your history that your heart problems developed after your son died. You said that you felt like your heart has been damaged by grief. I notice that you are Roman Catholic, and that you have been going to Mass every day since your son died. If you would like, I can arrange to have the priest come and visit you daily. We also have a person who helps clients who have recently lost a loved one. Would you like her to stop by?

14. As you explain treatments and procedures, use gestures and simple lay terms. Repeat key words. Avoid technical terminology. Say "your heart attack," not "your myocardial infarction."

15. Explain the steps of procedures in sequence and use progressive statements. "First, place the ice bag on your ankle for 20 minutes. Next, take the ice bag off of your ankle. One hour later, put the ice bag back on your ankle for another 20 minutes."

16. Use diagrams to explain procedures. Clients who are not literate may be confused by two-dimensional diagrams. In these cases, try to use a model if available. For example, use a model of the ear canal to explain how to self-administer ear drops.

17. Use props to demonstrate a procedure. Before giving an injection, first show the client the equipment (a syringe, needle, alcohol wipes), and then demonstrate how to give an injection. Have the client do a return demonstration. If the client has not grasped the procedure, go through the steps of the demonstration and repeat the demonstration again.

18. Observe how your client responds to your instructions. Does he say he understands what you want? Is she able to complete the steps of a procedure? Also, observe the person's body language. Does the client appear to be upset, confused, withdrawn, or embarrassed? If so, you will want to stop and explore how the client is feeling.

19. Involve the family in your teaching program. Ask one family member to act as a liaison to the client's extended family. List the name and phone number of that person in the client's room, chart, and care plan.

20. Make it easy for the client and family to contact you for information and instructions once the client goes home. If you are not able to act as a client contact, then arrange for another health care professional to do so.

21. Recognize that clients from diverse cultures may have legitimate reasons for not complying with your instructions. When clients do not comply, remember that their behavior may be perfectly consistent with cultural values that differ from yours and from the biomedical health care system. Clients who do not comply may also suffer from these problems:

    • Decisional conflict related to conflicting cultural values and beliefs.

    • Relocation stress syndrome related to cross-cultural migration.

    • Impaired verbal communication related to language barriers.

COMMUNICATION CONSIDERATIONS

*Never try to force change or demand **compliance** from clients. Instead, elicit information from clients that will help you arrive at a mutually agreed upon care plan and teaching plan. Decide which instructions clients must follow for reasons of safety, and then be prepared to negotiate on less crucial items.*

When instructing clients who do not speak English or who are not fluent in the language, you will want to perform the following steps in addition to the ones listed above.

1. Arrange for an interpreter to help you explain procedures and obtain consent.

2. Try to communicate with the client while you wait for the interpreter to arrive. Never ignore a client because he or she does not speak your language.

3. Ask a family member to provide additional help with interpreting prior to surgery or other important procedures. Allow family members to be in the postanesthesia room immediately after the client regains consciousness.

4. When instructing a client who does not speak English, frown when you want to signify that the client should not do something (e.g., no food now). Similarly, nod and smile when you want to reinforce a behavior. When you pour a glass of water, nod and smile as you place the glass in the client's hand, and then initiate the action of drinking a glass of water.

5. Do use picture cards or a phrase chart (use phonetic pronunciation) as you instruct your clients.

6. If you are caring for a child who does not understand English, you might try short phrases such as, "OK let's go." Try singing children's songs that may be familiar to the child. Use calming gestures and a soothing voice.

7. Assess for comprehension when relaying instructions. Do not assume that the client's nodding means the client understands.

8. Look for verbal and nonverbal exchanges between the client and the family (glances, shaking heads). Do these actions indicate understanding or lack of understanding?

9. Try to locate written educational materials that are in the language of the reader, and at the appropriate level of comprehension. For this step, you may need the aid of an interpreter.

The *Transcultural Communication Care Plan* that follows illustrates some of the transcultural communication techniques discussed in this chapter.

TRANSCULTURAL COMMUNICATION CARE PLAN

Communicating With A Hispanic Client With Heart Failure

Name: J. Gonzales

Age: 65

Physician: Dr. Grey

Medical Diagnosis Chronic heart failure

PROBLEM STATEMENT

Impaired verbal communication related to limited English proficiency.

ASSESSMENT

- Client speaks Spanish.
- Client speaks and understands a few basic words in English.
- Client's wife speaks and understands more English words than her husband, but is still very limited.
- Client says over and over. "No understand you, no understand you, no understand!"

Expected Outcomes	Interventions	Evaluation
1. Through the interpreter, client will be able to communicate his symptoms and health concerns.	1. Schedule an interpreter to assist with client assessment, treatments, and teaching/learning sessions.	1. Mr. Gonzales expressed his symptoms and learning needs through the interpreter.
2. With the aid of the interpreter, client will be able to give his informed consent to procedures and specify advance directives.	2. Have interpreter explain diagnostic and treatment procedures, informed consent forms, and advance directives.	2. Mr. Gonzales has signed an informed consent for diagnostic procedures. He also made out a living will.

(continued)

Expected Outcomes	Interventions	Evaluation
3. With aid of interpreter, client and wife will feel prepared to follow the prescribed medical regime at home, and will keep appointments for follow-up clinic visits.	3. Have interpreter assist with discharge planning and scheduling of follow-up clinic appointments.	3. Mr. Gonzales understands his medical regime. His wife has marked down the date in her calendar for their first follow-up clinic visit.

PROBLEM STATEMENT

Fluid volume excess related to knowledge deficit of low-sodium diet.

ASSESSMENT

- Peripheral edema and neck vein distention present.
- Client reports eating spicy Mexican foods at home.
- Client usually asks for salt to sprinkle on his hospital meals.
- Client says: "No salt? Why not?"

Expected Outcomes	Interventions	Evaluation
1. Client will be able to understand instructions and ask questions about the new diet.	1. Schedule learning sessions with client, wife, and interpreter.	1. Mr. Gonzales and wife asked many questions about the new diet.
2. Client will be able to explain why a low-sodium diet will help his heart condition.	2. Have interpreter explain to client why it is important to limit sodium intake.	2. Mr. Gonzales was able to explain the purpose of a low-sodium diet in his own words.
3. Client will be able to list the items that are not allowed on a low-sodium diet.	3. Discuss the foods, beverages, and seasonings that are not allowed on a low-sodium diet.	3. Mr. Gonzales was able to list the items that are not allowed on his low-sodium diet. He seemed to accept these dietary limitations.

(continued)

Expected Outcomes	Interventions	Evaluation
4. Client will be able to list the foods, beverages, and seasonings that are allowed on a low-sodium diet. He will find out where to purchase these items.	4. Discuss the foods, beverages, and seasonings that are allowed on a low-sodium diet. Explore where the client and wife can find these items when grocery shopping.	4. Mr. Gonzales was able to list the items that are on his diet. His wife knows where she can find these items in their local supermarket.
5. Client and wife will be able to modify client's favorite recipes to conform to a low-sodium diet without losing "taste appeal."	5. Schedule a meeting with the client, wife, dietitian, and interpreter. Have wife bring favorite recipes so that dietitian can modify them to conform with client's low-sodium diet.	5. Mr. Gonzales' wife brought the client's favorite recipes to the meeting. Mr. Gonzales told interpreter that he will stay on his new diet as long as he can eat his favorite foods, even though they might taste a little different.

PROBLEM STATEMENT

Nonadherence to clinic appointment schedule related to inability to access public or private transportation.

ASSESSMENT

- Client discharged from the hospital 3 weeks ago; has missed 3 clinic appointments.
- Client lives in a rural area that is 50 miles from the clinic.
- Client and wife do not own a car.
- Using public transportation requires several transfers, and is too exhausting for client.
- Client told interpreter: "I am just too tired to wait for all those buses, and too broke to buy a car."

Note: *This problem statement uses the term* **nonadherence** *rather than* **noncompliance**. *Nonadherence is less judgmental, and thus a more culturally appropriate health care problem statement.*

(continued)

Expected Outcomes	Interventions	Evaluation
1. Client and wife will be available for a home visit.	1. Arrange for a meeting at the client's home. Have client, wife, interpreter, and social service worker present.	1. Mr. and Mrs. Gonzales seemed glad to meet with us. Client has been experiencing symptoms of CHF, including orthopnea.
2. Client will understand that he must have follow-up medical care to control symptoms.	2. Have interpreter explain the importance of follow-up visits to clinic.	2. Mr. Gonzales told interpreter that he felt very badly about missing his clinic appointments, but he just could not find good transportation.
3. Client will adhere to the cabulance schedule, and be ready to go to the clinic for appointments.	3. Ask social services to look into having a cabulance pick client up on clinic days.	3. Mr. Gonzales said to go ahead and make the arrangements for a cabulance to pick him up for his appointments.
4. Client or his wife will let social services know if he is feeling too ill to go to the clinic.	4. Contact visiting nurse services. Arrange for home visits on days that client is not up to taking a cabulance to the clinic.	4. Mr. Gonzales was relieved to know that he would receive care at home on days that he was too ill to go into the clinic.
5. Client will keep clinic appointments once arrangements are made for cabulance.	5. Check with clinic to make sure Mr. Gonzales is keeping appointments.	5. Cabulance was arranged; Mr. Gonzales has kept his last 3 clinic appointments.

TESTING YOUR KNOWLEDGE

Circle the correct answer.

1. Select the communication technique that will help you to communicate most effectively with clients from other cultures.
   a. show interest by asking the client multiple questions
   b. listen, explain, and acknowledge differences
   c. reassure the client that everything will be all right
   d. give the client advice about health practices

2. In order to prepare a culturally appropriate care plan, you will need to assess
   a. the client's level of knowledge regarding the biomedical health care system.
   b. personal and community resources available to the client.
   c. cultural demands that compete with the client's attention to important health care needs.
   d. all of the above

3. Which of these activities describe what you should do when a client from another culture refuses to comply with important health care instructions?
   a. Warn the client about the consequences of failing to follow important health care instructions.
   b. Ask the physician to talk with the client about the failure to comply.
   c. Request that another health care professional work with the client.
   d. Fine tune your care plan so that it accommodates your client's cultural values and beliefs.

4. The Patient Self-Determination Act (PSDA) grants to clients which one of the following rights?
   a. the right to refuse treatment provided they have sufficient reason
   b. the right to refuse treatment without a reason
   c. the right to demand a specific medication or procedure that they believe will help them to recover
   d. the right to demand a specific medication or procedure and receive it, provided they agree to take responsibility for any complications

5. In this chapter, you read about Mr. Gonzales, a 65-year-old Hispanic male with congestive heart failure, who needed a low-sodium diet. From the following learning objectives, select the one for Mr. Gonzales that is most measurable:
   a. Mr. Gonzales will understand the reasons for his special diet.
   b. Mr. Gonzales will appreciate the number of low-sodium seasonings available for people on low-sodium diets.
   c. Mr. Gonzales will be able to list foods, seasonings, and beverages that are high in sodium and that are not allowed on his diet.
   d. Mr. Gonzales and his wife will be familiar with low-sodium foods.

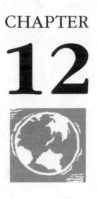
USING TRANSCULTURAL COMMUNICATION TO ASSIST PEOPLE RESPONDING TO PAIN, GRIEF, DYING, AND DEATH

Oneida M. Hughes, PhD, RN

KEY TERMS

- Appropriate Death
- Death-accepting
- Death-defying
- Death-denying
- Emotive
- Grief

- Grieving Process
- Pain Phenomenon
- Pain Perception
- Pain Responses
- Stoicism

OBJECTIVES

After completing this chapter, you should be able to:

- Describe the significance of using transcultural communication when caring for clients from diverse cultural backgrounds who are experiencing pain.

- Identify barriers to effective transcultural communication between health care professionals and family members whose loved one is dying.

- Describe two broad categories of responses to pain and characteristic features of each.

- Identify nonpharmacologic pain control measures that you can teach to clients to enhance their self control over the pain.

- Differentiate between different ethnic or cultural groups' responses to pain.

- Identify questions that you can use to elicit the client's perspective regarding pain.

- Explain three health care practice implications based on responses to pain for each cultural group: Hispanic Americans, Asian Americans, Black Americans, White Anglo Americans, and Native Americans.

- Differentiate between different ethnic/cultural groups' responses to death.

- Describe health care strategies that you can use to effectively assist persons who are grieving.

- Describe five principles that can guide health care professionals during grief counseling.

INTRODUCTION

Pain, dying, death, and grief are powerful universals that eventually affect all people, regardless of their land of birth, culture, or station in life. Although these events produce *similar* responses in people throughout the world (tears, moaning, sighing, screaming out), human responses also *vary*, depending on the person's culture. For example, Asian cultures tend to promote a stoical response to pain and grief, whereas black cultures usually allow emotional expressions of pain and grief. Health care professionals work intimately with clients and families who are experiencing pain, dying, death, and grief. To support people who are trying to cope with these stressful events, you will need to develop your transcultural communication skills.

To communicate effectively with clients from diverse cultures, it is important to understand the cultural bases for *why* clients and their families react as they do to pain, grief, dying and death. A lack of sensitivity concerning the effect of culture on a client's reactions can lead to poor communication, misinterpretation of symptoms, misdiagnoses, and faulty interventions. This chapter addresses how to use transcultural communication to assess, counsel, and console clients from diverse cultures who are suffering and who need your help.

USING TRANSCULTURAL COMMUNICATION TO ASSIST CLIENTS IN PAIN

Pain is a subjective sensation caused by noxious stimuli that signals actual or potential tissue damage. Pain is also a highly personal and private experience influenced by cultural learning, the meaning of the situation, and other factors unique to the individual (Hughes, 1997). An individual's definition of pain, like that of health and illness, is influenced by personal, social, and cultural experiences.

The Pain Phenomenon

Pain is a universally recognized **phenomenon** and an important area of consideration in health care delivery (Ludwig-Beymer, 1995; Hughes, 1997). Pain probably provides people with the most frequent and compelling reason for seeking health care.

Individuals and cultural groups vary in their **pain responses**. How people react to pain is influenced by their *perception* of pain. **Pain perception**, in turn, reflects each individual's attitude toward pain and characteristic way of responding to pain.

The point at which a sensation is first physically perceived and verbalized as painful is called the *pain threshold*. The maximum level of pain a person is willing to endure is called *pain tolerance*. Tolerance to pain is influenced by the individual's cultural background.

Expressions of pain also vary from culture to culture. What is appropriate verbal behavior and body language in response to pain is often dictated by culture. For example, the Japanese culture does not approve of loud verbal expressions of pain." Moreover, *within* each culture, expressions of pain may vary from person to person. For instance, how people express their pain is strongly influenced by their level of assimilation and acculturation into American culture. First and second generation immigrants are more likely to respond to pain in conventional ways that are accepted within their traditional culture (Zatnick & Dimsdale, 1990). On the other hand, later generations of immigrants who have assimilated the values of their new culture are less likely to retain traditional attitudes toward pain. There is also a wide range of responses among *subgroups* within the larger ethnic group. For this reason, never assume that all clients from a particular ethnic or cultural group will respond to pain in the same way.

Two broad categories of responses to pain are stoic and emotive responses (Salerno, 1995). Clients who are **stoic** in their response to pain are less expressive verbally and nonverbally, and they rarely complain.

Clients who are **emotive** will be quite vocal and will express their pain loudly.

Some reasons for a stoic response to pain include

1. denial of pain

2. a desire to be the perfect client

3. avoiding loss of control

4. avoiding worrying the family

5. fear of addiction

6. fear of overdose and side effects from pain medications

7. paying a price for past sins and future joys

8. acceptance of the pain.

Some reasons for an emotive response to pain include

1. fear of the pain

2. a desire for help and fear of not receiving it

3. anger

4. grief over loss of role and dignity

5. exorcism of the pain through the act of crying out

6. experiencing great pain.

In relation to gender, men demonstrate greater stoicism than women; however, research indicates that stoicism decreases with increasing age (Zatnick & Dimsdale, 1990).

Transcultural Differences in Responses to Pain

Mexican Americans are comprised of several diverse subcultural groups, including Hispanics, Puerto Ricans, Spanish Americans, Latin Americans, Latinos, and Chicanos. These different Mexican American subcultures tend to have their own sets of pain-related values, beliefs, and practices.

- Mexican Americans tend to view pain as a necessary part of life, and as an indicator of the seriousness of an illness. Mexican Americans believe that enduring sickness, including pain, is a sign of strength. Men often tolerate pain until it becomes unbearable (Klessig, 1992; Villarruel & de Montellano, 1992).

- Puerto Rican clients sometimes deny or avoid dealing with pain, but they may exhibit a high anxiety level. Some study findings revealed that Puerto Ricans demonstrated "greater expressiveness of pain, greater interference of pain with daily activities, and higher levels of emotional response to pain" (Gordon, 1997).

- Hispanics and Latin Americans tend not to verbalize complaints of pain.

Asian Americans are comprised of several highly diverse subcultures. In many Asian subcultural groups, pain is considered a serious symptom of illness for which biomedical care is sought. Acupuncture is a popular treatment for many health problems, including pain. Asians generally are quiet in voice and demeanor when in pain (Weber, 1996).

- Chinese culture values silence, "and women experiencing the pain of childbirth typically believe they will dishonor themselves and their families by a loud or wild response to pain" (Weber, 1996).

- Japanese Americans regard pain as an integral part of illness and traditionally exhibit a stoic attitude toward it. Some Japanese Americans feel that it is disgraceful to express pain verbally, even when their perception of the pain is intense. Clients may refuse pain medication when offered. Gordon (1997) reported that the Japanese tend to hide their pain under a stoic or unemotional demeanor. They may not readily "admit to being in pain and probably will not want to be touched as a comfort measure."

- Filipino Americans tend to view pain as "God's will for my life" and that neither the client nor physician should interfere with God's plan. Some Filipinos believe that illness may be attributed to a punishment from God and it would not be appropriate to interfere. Refusal of pain medication may be grounded in deep religious beliefs and should be respected. Some Filipino clients, especially the elderly, tend to hide their pain (Gordon, 1997; Kumasaka, 1996).

Black Americans form the largest minority cultural group in the United States. Recall from Chapter 2 that black American culture consists of several highly diverse subcultural groups. Depending on their cultural background, some black clients may deny or avoid dealing with pain until it is unbearable and then seek emergency care. Other blacks, who share mainstream attitudes about pain, may exhibit a stoic response to pain out of a desire to be a *perfect client*. Still other black clients may feel that an overt reaction to pain poses a threat to their self-esteem, and that denying the pain will be more acceptable to their caregivers. Black Americans with strong religious beliefs may believe that life on earth (with all of its pain and suffering), is only bearable because there will be happiness and lack of pain after death.

White, Anglo-Saxon, American culture, currently the dominant cultural group in America, is also comprised of many diverse subcultural groups from many countries. White Anglo Americans generally regard pain as a symptom of illness or injury. Evidence suggests that whites exhibit a moderate level of pain tolerance, express pain behavior more readily than blacks, and are more likely to seek pain relief. The majority of whites seek professional attention when their symptoms interfere with their vocation or avocational activity.

Native Americans are comprised of an estimated 300 Indian nations who reside mostly in the western part of the United States. Each Native American community has its own distinctive characteristic style of dealing with pain. However, in general, Native Americans are quiet in voice and demeanor, and they traditionally exhibit a stoic attitude and tolerate a high level of pain (Weber, 1996). Some clients may not seek pain relief and may tolerate pain until they are physically disabled.

Pain: Using Transcultural Communication to Plan Care

When clients are from other cultures, plan to use transcultural communication to assess pain, plan care, intervene with pain control measures, teach clients about pain interventions, and provide information about pain control. It is also important to talk with clients about their view of pain, previous pain control practices, their knowledge regarding the source or cause of the pain, and their preferences and expectations regarding pain relief. In addition, you should examine your own beliefs and values regarding pain, and demonstrate the importance you place on pain control by responding quickly and appropriately to relieve the client's pain.

Pain assessment, care planning and intervention is an on-going process. Reassessments and evaluation should also be continuous and on-going. It is important to thoroughly assess and document the client's physiologic reactions, verbal reports, and behavioral expressions of pain on a frequent basis.

COMMUNICATION CONSIDERATIONS

Remember that what the client says about the pain is the single most reliable indicator of the nature and intensity of the pain (United States Department of Health and Human Services Public Health Services, 1992).

Two general goals for pain management are to (1) eliminate or reduce the severity of the pain, and (2) enhance client comfort and satisfaction. An interdisciplinary health care team should plan specific pain control measures which include the client and family, when appropriate.

Both pharmacologic and nonpharmacologic therapies are used to control pain. You should evaluate the effects of drug and non-drug therapy on a frequent basis. You also need to encourage the client to let you know when pain is relieved or not relieved by specific therapies. Pain control therapy can then be readjusted on the basis of what the client says about the pain and pain relief.

COMMUNICATION CONSIDERATIONS

 When language is a barrier, arrange for an interpreter to assist in obtaining information about the client's pain, and in interpreting pain control strategies for the client.

Clients also need to learn about how to use nonpharmacologic pain control strategies. These strategies provide the client with self-control measures that may be used alone or in conjunction with pharmacologic measures to enhance pain relief. Teaching clients nonpharmacologic pain control measures will enhance their sense of control over the pain.

Some examples of nonpharmacologic pain strategies are (United States Department of Health and Human Services Public Health Services, 1992):

Cognitive-Behavioral	Physical Agents
• Education and instruction	• Heat or cold applications
• Relaxation	• Massage, exercise, immobilization
• Imagery	• Transcutaneous electrical
• Music distraction	nerve stimulation
• Biofeedback	

Melzack and Wall's (1965) *gate control theory of pain* provides the theoretical explanation for pain, and for the effectiveness of various pain control measures. The gate control theory suggests that a neutral system composed of a specialized body of cells in the dorsal horn of the spinal cord acts as a gating mechanism that blocks or decreases the transmission of pain stimuli to the higher brain centers. In addition, sensory stimuli from the higher brain centers (e.g., auditory and visual centers) and selective brain processes such as emotions and cognition, are able to transmit impulses that close the gate to incoming pain stimuli. (Walker, Tan, & George, 1995; Melzack & Wall, 1965).

The *chemical pain control theory* suggests that the body manufactures endogenous substances or endorphins that have analgesic properties. These endorphins act by binding to opioid receptors in the brain and spinal cord, and blocking the transmission of pain impulses.

Pain: Using Transcultural Communication to Explain, Counsel, and Console

Using transcultural communication is critically important when assessing, querying, teaching, and counseling clients from diverse cultures who are experiencing pain. To involve the client and family in setting goals and planning pain control strategies that are culturally acceptable, you can:

- Communicate openness, acceptance, and a willingness to listen to their views about pain and its control.

- Respect clients' autonomy by accepting choices they make about pain control. Allow mentally competent clients to retain some sense of control over their lives, including pain control.

- Be available to the client who is experiencing pain. Sitting with the client may decrease the person's anxiety level as well as pain level.

- Provide information about pain control in a clear manner, repeating important information.

- Provide information graphically to help reduce any language problem. For example, use a body line drawing when discussing specific areas of pain or discomfort, and use a numerical scale when discussing or evaluating pain intensity. Clients may require many teaching sessions to learn how to adequately care for themselves or family members.

- Secure a clergy member for the client if requested. Different ethnic and cultural groups derive solace and comfort from different spiritual sources.

- Listen to your clients' descriptions of their pain and the degree of pain relief.

- Seek the support of colleagues and health team members to assist you in exploring cultural specific pain management strategies.

USING TRANSCULTURAL COMMUNICATION TO ASSIST CLIENTS WHO ARE DYING

Death is an inevitable phenomenon that influences how one looks at life. Death also makes life seem more meaningful and poignant. It is the underlying reason that people aspire and strive to find meaning in life. Because death is universal, each culture has developed its own beliefs, mores, norms, standards, and restrictions regarding responses to dying and death.

The Death Phenomenon

Each society's teleological view of life influences its responses to death. Three general patterns of responses have been identified: *death-accepting, death-defying,* and *death-denying* (Rando, 1984).

1. **Death-accepting** is a common response in some primitive societies, such as the Fiji Islanders and Trobrianders. In these societies, death is viewed as inevitable and a natural part of the life cycle. Dying is one of the activities of daily living.

2. **Death-defying,** an earlier practice, was a common response in societies such as early Egypt.

3. **Death-denying** is an accepted response in the United States. Many Americans refuse to confront death, and try to protect themselves from the realities of death. Death is viewed as antithetical to living and not a normal part of human existence.

Transcultural Differences in Responses to Dying

Mexican Americans consider death as God's will. Mexican Americans' concept of death and an afterlife is deeply rooted in Roman Catholicism. They generally believe that enduring sickness is a sign of strength. When a client is terminally ill, the family is involved in all aspects of decision making.

Asian Americans have different views about death depending on their particular culture.

- *Chinese* culture holds bipolar views regarding death. One view is that death is only the vanishing of the human body; the true body exists forever. They believe that nature should be allowed to take its course, especially when a client is suffering. Chinese philosophy has long advocated the right to choose death. The second view is that life should be valued and preserved at all costs, and that health care professionals should do all within their power to save lives, even when the client is suffering from a painful and incurable disease (Corr, Nabe, & Corr, 1994).

- *Filipino Americans* tend to believe that people die because they have offended God or they are possessed by the spirit. They believe that dying is God's plan and that neither the client, nor physician, should interfere with God's will (Kumasaka, 1996).

- *Korean Americans'* traditional values dictate that clients should die at home.

Black Americans hold two belief systems regarding death (Jackson, 1980). The first belief system (based on the sacred norm) suggests that death provides an escape from this world, and that people should look for glory in the afterworld. The second belief system (based on the secular norm) suggests that black people view death as part of the normal life process and as an inevitable event. Death should also be accepted as a frequent companion. The secular norm assumes that death is a natural event, in spite of its highly disturbing social and emotional impact (Corr, Nabe, & Corr, 1994).

In many spirituals and in poetry written by black authors, the following themes are common: death as *freedom, rest, departure, finding peace, finding rest through closeness with Jesus,* and *death as a reward* (Corr, Nabe, & Corr, 1994).

White, Anglo Americans exhibit a wide array of emotions in response to the death of loved ones. Many respond to death with expressions of stoicism and a brave face rather than open expressions of grief. Spiritual beliefs and traditions vary across the subgroups. Many believe in immortality and place high value on family closeness (Pickett, 1993).

Native Americans view death as part of the life cycle: the old must die and the young may die. Although most conceive of life and death as circular, Native American cultures deal with death in different ways. For instance, burial practices vary among tribal groups. Many tribal groups hold long, somber wakes where food and memorial gifts are distributed. Some tribal groups mandate burying the deceased within 24 hours. Others forbid leaving the deceased alone and stipulate that a family member remain in attendance until the burial (Corr, Nabe, & Corr, 1994; Lawson, 1990).

Navajos fear death, and they distance themselves from death. Thus, Navajo clients often die in a hospital rather than at home. Navajos believe that clients with a terminal illness should be told that they may die. However, it is generally not acceptable to discuss death at length. Navajos respond to death and dying in a stoic manner. They are generally quiet in voice and demeanor. Navajos usually avoid touching the dead or dying person as well as items associated with death. Some Navajo health care professionals may have a healing ceremony performed after contact with a dead person.

COMMUNICATION CONSIDERATIONS

 The Navajo language does not always have words that are similar in meaning to English words. To communicate with Navajo-speaking clients and families, use interpreters who are fluent in the Navajo language.

The *Luguna Pueblos* perform a prescribed ritual for burying the dead. The death ritual may be in the form of chanting or monotonous singing over the dead to frighten away evil spirits. They do not permit the body to be taken to a mortuary, but perform the wrapping of the body themselves.

Dying: Using Transcultural Communication to Plan Care

Assisting clients to achieve an appropriate death requires effective transcultural communication and collaboration among clients, family members, and health care professionals. An **appropriate death** has been defined as a death one might choose, given the choice (Picket, 1993). The essential components of an appropriate death are symptom control, comfort, and support. Showing respect for clients and family members, and encouraging their active participation in decisions related to the client's final days should guide your plan of care.

To help people from different cultures express their loss and grief in ways that are valued in their culture, you need to first clarify your own values and feelings about death, loss, and grief. Health care professionals who are consciously aware of their own values and preferences will be less likely to practice *cultural imposition*, which is the tendency to impose ones beliefs, values, and patterns of behavior upon clients from other cultures.

COMMUNICATION CONSIDERATIONS

 It is critical that health care professionals recognize, understand, and respect each client's and family's cultural specific values regarding dying and death.

Different cultures have different needs when confronted with dying and death. *Mexican Americans* view the nuclear and extended family as vitally important. The immediate and extended family is a "primary source of social support, tangible aid, information, and advice," therefore, "directing services toward the entire family is absolutely essential." Close friends are also primary sources of social support. It is important to provide family and friends with tangible aid, information, and advice.

Traditionally, the father or husband is the head of the Mexican household, and may make all major decisions regarding the dying loved one. Mexican Americans who are separated from family and other contacts may feel a sense of isolation when faced with a dying child or relative, and consequently they are more likely to need the support of health team members.

Mexican Americans consider death to be God's will, a belief that is rooted in their religious heritage. They are very expressive in emotions and behavior. Mexican Americans may wish to have a priest present when a person is dying to perform last rites (Corr, Nabe, & Corr, 1994). Kind words and a gentle touch from health care professionals convey a sense of caring, which will help to comfort the dying client.

Asian Americans are very family oriented. The extended family should be involved in the care of the dying client, as family members provide social support, resources and tangible aid. Remember to incorporate relevant cultural values when planning care for the dying client who is Asian. For example, Asian Americans have a deep respect for the body. Asians may feel that the body is not their own possession, but is passed down from their ancestors. Some Asians believe that the head is sacred and they consider it disrespectful to touch the head without permission. They may also consider it disrespectful to make direct eye contact.

When planning care for the dying client, health care professionals must remember that many Asian and Islamic women are afraid of being examined by a male. They prefer being examined by a female whenever possible. When they are examined by a male, the unnecessary removal of underclothing should be avoided, and a female should be in attendance.

COMMUNICATION CONSIDERATIONS

When communicating and interacting with the dying client's family, remember that smiling and nodding do not necessarily reflect understanding or agreement. Actually for many Asians, smiling and nodding are signs of respect.

Many Asians feel that a sick person should never be left alone. This need may be accommodated by allowing family members to remain with the dying client at all times.

Black Americans are also family oriented, and the extended family is very important. It is customary for many family members to remain with a dying client in the hospital. Although the family is central, friends and church members also provide support and comfort as they visit often and pray for the client (Corr, Nabe, & Corr, 1994). Expressions of grief for the dying client may include crying, screaming, and various other emotions and behaviors. Health care professionals should involve the client and family when planning and implementing care.

White, Anglo Americans, as a death-denying culture, may try to cheat death by using extraordinary measures to save lives, even when clients are clearly suffering and dying. The strong need by some health care professionals and medical personnel to prolong life at any cost is an example of a death-denying attitude. Even when death comes after a long and difficult illness, it seems to be the *American way* to restrain expressions of grief, and face the death of loved ones with quiet stoicism. Most white Americans do value their families, and family closeness does provide a source of support when a family member is dying. Because middle-class Americans also value self-determination, it is important to involve the dying client and the family in all aspects of decision-making and care planning.

Native Americans view the family, both nuclear and extended, as being highly important. Being there for a dying family member is of prime importance. Ross (1981) reports that "many Native-Americans believe that the spirit of a dying person cannot leave the body until the family is there." It is not unusual for many members of the extended family to remain with the dying client, in close proximity, until death has occurred (Lawson, 1990). For instance, restrictive hospital rules have no meaning for Navajo people, and they may resist leaving the dying client's bedside just because "Visiting hours are over."

When planning care for the dying Native American client, it is best to obtain information by listening to rather than by directly interviewing family members. Some Native Americans feel that talking about their dying loved one detracts from the spiritual context and may bring bad luck. In addition, Native Americans may refuse to answer questions because they are suspicious of people of European descent. However, you may be able to overcome the family's initial reluctance to talk with you by showing respect and being sensitive to their point of view (Lawson, 1990).

Dying: Using Transcultural Communication to Explain, Counsel, and Console

There are several important ways to help clients and families cope with the process of dying.

1. Help the family identify resources within their church or community to which they can turn for comfort and solace.

2. Recognize that members of different cultures need different types of support from their health care professionals. Explain to the client and family what types of help the hospital and community can provide.

3. Demonstrate a willingness to listen to the client's and family's fears and concerns. Help the client and family identify inner strengths or religious beliefs that will allow them to emotionally cope with the trauma of facing death.

4. Recognize that the family system is very important in most cultural groups. Always consider the family as a unit when planning care for a loved one who is dying. Evaluate how the family structure influences the client's response to dying, as well as the family's role in providing solace and support. Facilitate transcultural communication by showing your respect for family members and including them in your plan of care.

5. Serve as an advocate for the client and family by supporting cultural values that are important to them. For instance, allow clients to use traditional practices, including healers, if that is their wish.

USING TRANSCULTURAL COMMUNICATION TO ASSIST PEOPLE WHO ARE GRIEVING

Grief is a reaction that encompasses a broad range of feelings and behaviors that are associated with loss. It is a dynamic, pervasive process that occurs in phases, over time.

The Grieving Process

Expressions of grief vary from person to person, but they are almost always influenced by a person's ethnic and cultural background. *Thought patterns* that are commonly associated with the grieving process include:

- Disbelief
- Confusion
- Preoccupation
- Hallucinations

Behaviors that are frequently associated with grief reactions include:

- Sleep disturbances
- Appetite disturbances
- Absent-minded behavior
- Social withdrawal
- Distressing dreams
- Restlessness
- Crying
- Treasuring objects of the loved one

Transcultural Differences in Response to Grief

Providing grief support to individuals and family members requires compassion, understanding, and acceptance of how cultural traditions influence the grieving process. *Mexican Americans* perceive death to be God's will, and the culture dictates open expressions of grief. Religious practices such as praying for the dead and saying the rosary are significant aspects of the grieving process. The family is a source of support. Family members will need time and a private room where they can openly express their grief.

Asian Americans encompass many diverse cultural groups, with many different grieving patterns. Chinese are not publicly expressive of grief; however, some Chinese will feel comfortable venting their feelings, even when in public. Religious traditions are particularly important during stressful times. Japanese Americans respond to grief with denial or repression of emotions, which is an integral part of their culture. Because disclosure of feelings is viewed as bad manners, Japanese people are likely to be stoic when grieving (Corr, Nabe, & Corr, 1994; Pickett, 1993).

Black Americans may express their grief by crying and sometimes screaming; praying, singing, and reading scriptures. The family, minister, and friends are major sources of support. Black Americans should be allowed the time and a private area where they can express their grief (Corr, Nabe, & Corr, 1994).

White, Anglo Americans typically respond to grief with stoiscism and restrained emotions. However, expressions of sadness and the demonstration of emotions vary among white Americans. Family closeness and their religious traditions are significant sources of support (Ross, 1981).

Native Americans may or may not express grief publicly. However, they may fully express their emotions if they are in a sympathetic environment. Grief tends to be family oriented, with all members assuming roles in the grieving process.

Grief: Using Transcultural Communication to Plan Care

Cultural assessment provides the basis for planning culturally specific care for grieving family members. Transcultural communication helps to facilitate assessment and collaborative planning, as well as the development and refinement of intervention strategies that can be used to support grieving families. The cultural assessment should include data such as the family's ethnic or racial identity, value orientation, language or dialect, and family structure. This data can be used to plan culturally specific care.

COMMUNICATION CONSIDERATIONS

 As you perform your assessment and plan care, use an unhurried approach to show respect, compassion, and sensitivity for grieving family members.

Grief: Using Transcultural Communication to Explain, Counsel, and Console

You can help family members with the grieving process by following these steps.

1. Assist family members in dealing with their loss. Encourage each person to talk about the loss. Be a patient and active listener.

COMMUNICATION CONSIDERATIONS

 Working with grieving families whose native language is not English will require an interpreter, not only for exchanging information, but also for understanding finer shades of meaning.

2. Assist the person in identifying and expressing feelings such as anger, anxiety, guilt, and helplessness. Family members may not want to discuss certain feelings because they are upsetting and unpleasant. Feelings that are left unexpressed may go unresolved for long periods of time or even permanently.

3. Provide the family with time to grieve. Allow the family to start coming to terms with their loss and all of its ramifications. Remind the family that grieving is a process that occurs in phases, over time. Sometimes, grieving family members and friends are eager to get over the loss and its pain, and move back into a normal routine before they are ready.

4. Recognize that some points in time may be more difficult for the bereaved than others, such as the first anniversary of the death, or certain holidays. One effective intervention is to help the person anticipate this problem and prepare for it in advance.

5. Allow for individual as well as cultural differences. There is a wide range of behavioral responses to grief. Do not expect all family members who are grieving to grieve in the same way.

6. Help the person examine their defenses and coping styles. Some of the defenses and coping styles indicate competent behaviors; others do not. For example, a person who copes by using alcohol or drugs excessively is probably not making an effective adjustment to the loss. This person should be helped to explore other coping strategies.

7. Provide continuing support as necessary. Some people require continuing support over a long period of time. One way to offer continuing support is through support groups. There are special groups for those who have lost spouses, children, parents, and other loved ones. There are also groups within each culture that offer help and comfort to the bereaved. It is important to be aware of community and cultural resources, and make referrals, when necessary.

TESTING YOUR KNOWLEDGE

Circle the correct answer.

1. When assessing a client's pain, the health care professional must be cognizant that the single most reliable source of information is the
   a. client's report of their perception of pain.
   b. physician's perception of the client's pain.
   c. health care professional's perception of the client's pain.
   d. ethnic and cultural group's general views about pain.

2. The point at which a sensation is first physically perceived and verbalized is called
   a. pain perception.
   b. pain threshold.
   c. pain tolerance.
   d. pain reaction.

3. Each society's teleological views about life influence its response to death. The general pattern of responses to death in the United States is characterized as
   a. death-accepting.
   b. death-defying.
   c. death-denying.
   d. death-endearing.

4. Which cultural group is more likely to call for a priest when a person is dying?
   a. Native Americans
   b. Mexican Americans
   c. Black Americans
   d. Asian Americans

5. Which ethnic or cultural group may not easily admit to being in pain, and most likely will not want to be touched as a comfort measure?
   a. Native Americans
   b. Japanese Americans
   c. Hispanic Americans
   d. African Americans

6. Which ethnic or cultural group tends to feel that enduring pain is a part of life and a sign of strength?
   a. Native Americans
   b. Puerto Ricans
   c. Mexican Americans
   d. Black Americans

7. A death that one might choose, given the chance, is called
   a. good death.
   b. appropriate death.
   c. painless death.
   d. optimal death.

UNIT FOUR
EVALUATION

EVALUATING YOUR TRANSCULTURAL COMMUNICATION SKILLS IN PLANNING AND IMPLEMENTING CARE

The following exercises highlight some of the concepts that we discussed in this Unit. Make a note if you are selecting a different option than you would have *prior* to studying Chapters 11 and 12.

Exercise One: Evaluating How Comfortable You Feel When Planning and Implementing Care for Clients From Diverse Cultures

Recall that you performed this exercise before you began your study of this Unit. By now you should have read Chapters 11 and 12. You may also have had some new experiences in planning care, client teaching, providing pain relief, and assisting dying clients and grieving relatives.

The following statements contain assignments that you may have received as you cared for clients from diverse cultures. Using the following five levels of comfort, rate how comfortable you *now* feel about performing each assignment. Compare your current levels of comfort with your earlier levels.

- Level 1: I feel very uncomfortable.
- Level 2: I feel rather uncomfortable.
- Level 3: I feel fairly comfortable.
- Level 4: I feel comfortable.
- Level 5: I feel very comfortable.

1. *Assignment:* Talk with a client about his financial and home situation—two factors that can influence your plan of care. **1 2 3 4 5**

2. *Assignment:* Explain to a Japanese client who regularly uses soy sauce and other similar flavorings that he must reduce the sodium in his diet to control his congestive heart failure. **1 2 3 4 5**

247

3. *Assignment:* Negotiate a biomedical plan of care with a client from a culture that does not totally accept biomedical practices.

1 2 3 4 5

4. *Assignment:* Witness a client's signing of an *Informed Consent* prior to a major procedure. **1 2 3 4 5**

5. *Assignment:* Develop clear, realistic, and measurable learning objectives for a client who needs to learn about his medications, diet, rest, and activity schedule before going home. **1 2 3 4 5**

6. *Assignment:* Teach a client a procedure such as changing a dressing or self-administration of insulin. **1 2 3 4 5**

7. *Assignment:* Work closely with an interpreter to teach a client with limited English proficiency about his diet and medications.

1 2 3 4 5

8. *Assignment:* Counsel a client with chronic pain who is from a more emotive culture; for example, the Italian culture. **1 2 3 4 5**

9. *Assignment:* Counsel and console a dying client and his family who are observing cultural and religious rituals with which you are unfamiliar. **1 2 3 4 5**

Exercise Two: Evaluating Your Point of View Toward Transcultural Situations That Involve Planning, Teaching, Counseling, and Consoling

You also performed this exercise earlier in the self-assessment section of this Unit. Select the answers that best describe your point of view *now* that you have completed the chapters in this Unit. There is no scoring for these questions.

1. When planning care for clients from diverse cultures, you should
   a. make every effort to preserve the client's cultural practices.
   b. consider the client's cultural practices, but make the biomedical aspects of the client's care plan your major priority.
   c. convince the client that he should follow the biomedical care plan for his own good.
   d. let the client manage his own care as much as possible.

2. A client who refuses to follow a biomedical plan of care
   a. needs to have logical reasons for his refusal to follow the plan.
   b. is being unreasonable and noncompliant.
   c. is observing his legal and constitutional rights.
   d. is recklessly endangering his health, and should be scheduled for a psychiatric consult.

3. When teaching clients from diverse cultures:
   a. I try to provide the same information in the same way, regardless of the client's cultural background.
   b. I try to consider the client's special learning needs and limitations that are related to his culture or lack of proficiency in English.
   c. I don't believe that is possible to write measurable learning objectives for clients.
   d. I realize that sometimes it is necessary to negotiate with the client, and adapt my teaching plan to his cultural views and daily patterns.

4. When caring for clients from diverse cultures who are experiencing pain:
   a. I realize that some clients are more stoic in their response to pain, while other clients are more emotive.
   b. It is difficult to evaluate a client's pain when the person responds in a stoic manner, and refuses to acknowledge that the pain exists.
   c. It is difficult to work with clients who scream and cry when in pain.
   d. The client's own description of his or her pain is often inaccurate.

5. When caring for clients from diverse cultures who are dying:
   a. I try to accept the client's cultural values and behavior patterns regarding dying and death.
   b. I find it difficult to deal with the dying client's family when their continuous presence makes it hard for me to provide care.
   c. I don't know what to say when family members express their grief to me following the client's death.
   d. I don't feel that I have the experience to counsel a bereaved family from another culture.

Exercise Three: Reviewing Your *Transcultural Interaction Diary*

1. Have you had an opportunity to write a care plan or a teaching plan for a client from another culture? _____

2. How did your client react to your plan? Did the person find the plan acceptable, partially acceptable, or unacceptable due to his or her cultural beliefs? _____

   _____

3. If partially acceptable or unacceptable, what did you do or say to negotiate with the client? _____

   _____

Were you able to reach a satisfactory compromise with the client?

_____

If you were unable to reach a compromise, were you able to accept the client's decisions regarding his or her own care and learning needs?

_____

4. What teaching methods have you been using when instructing clients about their care? _____

_____

Which method do you feel most comfortable with? _____

Have you been able to follow a client's progress following discharge?

_____

Has the client continued to follow your instructions?

_____

5. How do you plan to improve your teaching plans and activities?

_____

_____

6. Have you had an opportunity to assess clients from other cultures who responded stoically to pain? _____

What did you do to assess the client?

_____

_____

What did you do to relieve the client's pain?

_____

_____

7. Have you had an opportunity to assess clients from other cultures who responded emotionally to pain? _____

What communication techniques did you use to assess the client?

_____

_____

What did you do to relieve the client's pain?

_____

_____

8. Have you been assigned a client from another culture who is dying?

_____

What religious and cultural practices did the client and family observe?

_____

_____

How did you feel about these practices? Comfortable or uncomfortable?

_____

9. What did you say and do to comfort the client? _____

_____

_____

What did you say and do to console the grieving family? _____

_____

_____

10. What can you do to improve your transcultural communication in situations that involve dying, death, and grieving?_____

_____

_____

Exercise Four: Evaluating Your Knowledge of Transcultural Communication Principles That Are Related to Planning and Implementing Care

Write a brief response to these questions, which are drawn from topics discussed in Chapters 11 and 12.

1. In general, developing a care plan involves four steps:
   a. _____
   b. _____
   c. _____
   d. _____

2. Madeline Leininger recommends the following three approaches when planning care for clients from diverse cultures:
   a. _____
   b. _____
   c. _____

3. The Patient Self-Determination Act (PSDA) guarantees clients the right to:

_____

_____

4. The five steps of the teaching/learning process are:

a. _____

b. _____

c. _____

d. _____

e. _____

5. Learning styles vary for clients from diverse cultures. Four types of learning styles include:

a. _____

b. _____

c. _____

d. _____

6. The five major steps of the *LEARN model* developed by Berlin and Folkes are:

a. _____

b. _____

c. _____

d. _____

e. _____

7. Five steps that are involved in teaching procedures to clients from diverse cultures are:

a. _____

b. _____

c. _____

d. _____

e. _____

8. Pain is defined as: _____

_____

9. Members of different cultural groups tend to respond to pain in different ways. Mexican Americans tend to view pain as: _____

_____

Asian Americans tend to view pain as: _____

_____

Black Americans tend to view pain as: _____

_____

White, Anglo-Saxon Americans tend to view pain as: _____

_____

Native Americans tend to view pain as: _____

_____

10. Describe six ways to use transcultural communication to plan care for clients who are in pain:
    a. _____
    b. _____
    c. _____
    d. _____
    e. _____
    f. _____

11. Three general patterns of responses to death are:
    a. _____
    b. _____
    c. _____

12. Describe five ways you can use transcultural communication to advise, counsel, and console people from diverse cultures who are going through the death experience:
    a. _____
    b. _____
    c. _____
    d. _____
    e. _____

13. Thought patterns associated with the grieving process include:

    _____

    _____

14. Behaviors associated with the grieving process include:

    _____

    _____

15. Describe seven ways you can use transcultural communication to advise, counsel, and console people from diverse cultures who are grieving:

a. _____

b. _____

c. _____

d. _____

e. _____

f. _____

g. _____

UNIT FIVE

TRANSCULTURAL COMMUNICATION SKILLS BETWEEN HEALTH CARE PROFESSIONALS

UNIT FIVE ASSESSMENT

ASSESSING YOUR TRANSCULTURAL COMMUNICATION SKILLS WITH OTHER HEALTH CARE PROFESSIONALS

Exercise One: Assessing your Personal Objectives

Up until now, you have primarily studied how to communicate with clients from other cultures. This Unit discusses barriers to transcultural communication between health care professionals, and presents techniques for overcoming those barriers.

What do *you* want to gain from studying this Unit? Check those points in the following list that apply to you, and also write down any other objectives.

My personal objectives are to:

_____ Learn how to relate better to staff members or health care students who are from other cultures.

_____ Identify and overcome biases and prejudices that are hindering me from working successfully with health care professionals from other cultures.

_____ Sharpen my skills in supervising ancillary personnel from diverse cultures.

_____ Decrease the frustration I feel when working with physicians or health care professionals who are not proficient in English, or who have strong accents.

_____ Welcome working with skilled foreign health care professionals, and appreciate the wealth of knowledge concerning other cultures that I can gain from them.

_____ Learn more about how to manage a diverse health care staff.

_____ Learn about how conflicts are resolved in the workplace.

My other personal objectives for learning how to communicate in a diverse workplace are to:

1. _____

2. _____

3. _____

256

4. _____

5. _____

Exercise Two: Assessing Your Personal Responses to Working With Health Care Professionals From Different Cultures

In today's diverse workplace, you will need to work closely with registered nurses, physicians, health care professionals and ancillary personnel who are from different cultures, and who speak English as a second language. How do you *really feel* about working with professionals who are from foreign countries, or from different racial or ethnic groups? Take a minute to answer the following questions. You do not need to share your answers with anyone, so be honest with yourself.

	Agree	Neutral	Disagree
I would rather work with American health care professionals than a foreign professional.	____	____	____
I find it frustrating to work with health care professionals who are not proficient in English.	____	____	____
If I thought that a health care professional was not fulfilling duties due to cultural or language problems, I would hesitate to report them for fear that I would be considered prejudiced.	____	____	____
I enjoy working with skilled foreign health care professionals. I feel that I can learn a lot from them.	____	____	____
I like to attend classes and informal meetings where I can learn more about how health care professionals from other countries are educated.	____	____	____
I do not feel prepared to work with or supervise an unlicensed assistive worker who has some problems with understanding English.	____	____	____

Exercise Three: Your *Transcultural Interaction Diary*

1. In Unit One, you set up and started your *Transcultural Interaction Diary*. Since then, you have been primarily recording your transcultural interactions with clients, families, and interpreters.

2. Today, set up a new section in your diary for recording significant transcultural interactions with supervising professionals, staff nurses, physicians, unlicensed assistive personnel, and other students.

3. Start using your diary now, before reading this chapter. Try to remember and record any past interactions that were either very positive or very negative. For each interaction, write down both the verbal and nonverbal transcultural communications that passed between you and the other health care professioanls. Record the feelings and thoughts that you had during and after each interaction.

4. Continue to keep your diary as you study this chapter. Try to use the various suggestions from the chapter for improving your transcultural communication with health professionals from different cultures. Note how using a particular technique helped to clarify your communications.

5. Remember to keep your diary in a private place. You will not feel as free to write about your positive and negative transcultural interactions with staff members if other people might read your personal experiences.

CHAPTER

13

FOSTERING TRANSCULTURAL COMMUNICATION WITH OTHER HEALTH CARE PROFESSIONALS

KEY TERMS

- Arbitration
- Collectivism
- Conflict Resolution
- External Locus of Control
- Individualism
- Internal Locus of Control

- Mediation
- Negotiation
- Perceived Injurious Experience
- Unperceived Injurious Experience

OBJECTIVES

After completing this chapter, you should be able to:

- Discuss the major barriers that impede transcultural communication between health care professionals from different cultures.
- Distinguish between the values of individualism and collectivism in the workplace, and give an example of each.
- Identify at least 10 different approaches that you can use to improve your transcultural communication with co-workers and ancillary personnel.

- Identify strategies that a health care manager can use to improve transcultural communication in the workplace.
- Discuss the dynamics of transcultural conflict in the workplace, and describe alternative methods for resolving workplace disputes.

INTRODUCTION

In addition to bridging the transcultural gap between themselves and their clients, health care professionals must also learn how to communicate with medical personnel from around the globe. The health care workforce of today is dramatically different from the workforce of the past. Over the last decade, large urban hospitals (primarily on the East and West Coasts and in the Sun Belt) have recruited foreign health care professionals to meet staffing demands (Williams & Rodgers, 1993). Moreover, the improved work and economic conditions in this country have attracted foreign professionals, primarily from the Philippines, Great Britain, Ireland, and Canada. In addition, the demand for ancillary personnel has increased the number of foreign workers and ethnically diverse minorities in the health care workplace. Unlicensed ancillary workers are expected to be the fastest growing health care occupational group into the 21st century (Sherer, 1993).

A multicultural health care workforce can have a positive effect on client care. Health care professionals from diverse backgrounds bring a variety of experiences and a wide range of knowledge to the health care setting. Health care professionals who are from different cultures offer fresh ideas and different solutions to long-term problems. Foreign professionals can help American professionals understand and relate better to clients who are also from diverse cultural backgrounds.

On the other hand, the cultural diversity of the workforce may raise barriers that can produce serious workplace problems. Foreign health care professionals are usually competent and committed workers, but nevertheless, daily interactions with native English-speaking health care professionals can be strained. American health care professionals may feel that foreign health care professionals are not as technically proficient as health care professionals educated in the United States. Furthermore, some foreign professionals come to the United States with their own biases, and they may feel that American health care professionals lack competence and compassion. In addition, ancillary personnel from diverse backgrounds may misunderstand and resent the white American health care professionals who are in charge.

The major barriers to transcultural communication between staff members, the resulting conflicts, and some possible solutions and resolutions are presented in the sections that follow.

BARRIERS TO TRANSCULTURAL COMMUNICATION BETWEEN HEALTH CARE PROFESSIONALS

Barriers to transcultural communication between health care professionals extend from confused pronouns and foreign terminology, to different values that result in different health care delivery styles. Major barriers are:

- Different cultural patterns and biases that affect the relationships between health care professionals
- Racism and prejudice that can undermine professional relationships.
- Clashes in values that arise between foreign health care professionals and health care professionals trained in the United States.
- Different perceptions of responsibilities and client care that are based on different cultural values.
- Differences in time orientation.
- Different systems of health care and medical education.
- Language differences that result in serious miscommunications.

Other factors that may affect the attitudes and performance of health care professionals from different cultures are:

1. the status of men, women, physicians, and health care professionals in the culture
2. attitudes toward authority figures
3. methods for financing health care
4. responsibilities of the client's family for providing health care
5. the use of artificial life-support systems
6. the perception of time as past-oriented, present-oriented, or future-oriented
7. the value of work as a health care professional (Lajkowicz, 1993).

Different Cultural Patterns and Biases

Cultural patterns and biases that staff members bring to the hospital can complicate communications, and create misunderstandings and resentments. For example, many male physicians from the Middle East think of women as subservient. These physicians may feel that they have the right to shout at female health care professionals and demand assistance from them. American health care professionals, who have been raised to think of themselves as equal to men, may be upset by the physicians' tone of voice and condescending manner. American health care professionals also can become frustrated by the lack of discussion, information sharing, and teamwork that often characterizes their relationships with physicians from the Middle East (Burner, 1990).

On the other hand, health care professionals from cultures that raise women to be subservient, may find it difficult to be assertive when working with American health care professionals and physicians. For example, if a Japanese born health care professional does not agree with an order from a physician, she may follow the order without protest, providing the order is not harmful to the client. In contrast, an American health care professional who does not agree with the physician's order may challenge the order, and argue with the physician. The Japanese health care professional raised in the traditional Japanese culture may regard the American health care professional as disrespectful of authority, and guilty of causing the physician to "lose face."

Racism and Prejudice

Chapter 4 introduced the concept that racism exists in the American health care delivery system as a formidable barrier that severely undermines transcultural communication. According to Barbee (1993), there are certain attributes of health care professionals that prevent individuals from openly confronting the racism that exists in their profession. These attributes are:

- *An emphasis on empathy.* Health care professionals perceive themselves as caring individuals who see all people as the same rather than different. Health care professionals are taught that illness has no color, and that their vocation is to help sick people, regardless of their color, creed, or race. This perception of themselves as caring makes it very difficult for health care professionals to acknowledge that they are capable of racism.

- *An individual orientation.* The major concepts that health care professionals learn in school are individualistic rather than group-oriented. Although health care delivery seems to emphasize families, groups, and communities, health care practice is geared to the needs of individuals. Also, schools of health care require students to study the hard sciences such as chemistry and physics, whereas social sciences such as sociology and anthropology are usually electives. As a consequence, health care students fail to learn enough about cultural diversity, and the multicultural milieu in which they will be working.

- *A preference for homogeneity and a need to avoid conflict.* According to Brink (1990), selection committees on health care faculties prefer a homogenous student body because it tends to be more efficient, non-challenging, and nonthreatening. Such characteristics reduce conflict and promote solidarity within the health care ranks.

These attributes have allowed the following three types of racism to flourish in American health care (Barbee, 1993):

1. *Denial.* There are several ways by which health care professionals can deny racism. Health care professionals—black and white—may simply refuse to use the term *race* or *racism*. Black health care professionals may believe that their humanitarian work makes them immune to racism, and thus for them racism does not exist. White health care professionals may substitute the more benign terms of *ethnocentrism, cultural bias,* and *cultural diversity* for the politically incorrect term of *racism,* thereby denying its existence.

2. *Color-blind perspective.* Health care professionals who adhere to the color-blind perspective believe that race is a social category that has no relevance to an individual's behavior, and thus "individuals should not notice each other's racial group membership" (Barbee, 1993). For those who adopt the color-blind perspective, race is a taboo topic, and they view social relationships as interpersonal rather than intergroup relationships.

   The color-blind perspective helps health care professionals to (a) avoid overt conflict with people of other races, (b) minimize the discomfort and embarrassment that is associated with discussions of race and racism, (c) ignore or distort the fact that cultural differences exist, and (d) protect themselves from charges of discrimination in the workplace.

3. *Aversive racism.* According to Barbee (1993), "aversive racism is characterized by ambivalence: feelings and beliefs associated with an egalitarian value system conflict with unacknowledged negative feelings and beliefs concerning blacks." This form of racism is subtle because aversive racists do not see themselves as prejudiced or discriminatory in any way.

   Although racism distorts transcultural communication, prejudices between the nationalities, social classes, and sexes *within a culture* can also cause communication problems. For example, prejudices within the Hispanic culture may make professionals from the Dominican Republic reluctant to work with Puerto Ricans. Second-generation Mexican-American health care professionals may not want to take orders from Central-American health care professionals or physicians. Some black men object to working for black women. Some Latin men refuse to take directions from Latin or black women (Burner, 1990).

Different Value Systems

Different value systems can also complicate transcultural communication between staff members. Health care professionals from different cultures may have:

1. different perceptions of staff responsibilities to each other
2. different perceptions of client care
3. a different locus of control.

Different Perceptions of Staff Responsibilities. Recall from Chapter Two that cultural values deeply influence what a person feels is most important: the welfare of the individual or the welfare of the group. **Individualism** emphasizes the importance of individual rights and rewards. **Collectivism** emphasizes the importance of group decisions, and places the rights of the group as a whole above the rights of any individual in the group.

> **Example:** Unlike Western health care professionals, Asian health care professionals tend to accept difficult assignments without complaint. They also may be more willing to do what American health care professionals might consider demeaning (e.g., cleaning cabinets).
>
> Because many Asian health care professionals value *the group,* they believe that an individual's duties have less value than the combined work of all of the health care staff on the unit.

Also, when assigned to difficult or menial tasks, health care professionals from Asian cultures may feel it is inappropriate to confront a supervisor and demand a change of assignment. Maintaining face and assuring harmony are Eastern cultural values that may be more important to Asian health care professionals than upsetting their supervisor in order to get an easier assignment. Indeed, an emphasis on minimizing conflict and commitment to group loyalty typify most Asian cultures.

In contrast, health care professionals educated in Western culture generally place more value on individualism and independence. Thus Western health care professionals may complain to the supervisor if they feel assignments are unfair or involve menial work. This assertive behavior is consistent with ingrained values of equitable work distribution, and the respect for education and professionalism that defines the American work style.

Western health care professionals also want to be *individually* recognized for their work; for instance they may want a promotion, or they may dream of being publicly honored for giving outstanding client care or other accomplishments.

Different Perceptions of the Health Care Professional's Role.
Health care professionals from different cultures have different perceptions of the health care professional's role and health care values, which American health care professionals may not appreciate.

> **Example:** in a study of Philippine-American nurses, the most important finding was the theme of *obligation to care* that prevailed in all aspects of their work (Spangler, 1992). This theme, which epitomized the Philippine-American nurses values, was expressed in three important ways:
>
> 1. ***Expressed seriousness and dedication to work.*** These nurses felt a strong sense of duty toward their clients, which was fully developed during their years in nursing school.
>
> 2. ***Attentiveness to the client's physical comfort needs.*** In the words of one nurse:
>
> > To me, it is very important that patients are physically comfortable. I clean them up.... I talk to them while I attend to their physical needs. With our busy schedule, this is the best time to get to know the patients.
>
> In contrast, mainstream American nurses tended to devalue the physical care of clients because of its association with the body and body products. Indeed, some American nurses regarded the physical care of clients as menial work. According to one Philippine-American nurse, "Here in the United States, the prestige is when you are away from the bedside; actual patient care is relegated to nurse's aides."
>
> 3. ***Respect and patience.*** The Philippine cultural values of respect and patience were learned early in life by the nurses, and were carried forth into their relationships with clients. As expressed by a Philippine-American nurse:

> We are very patient people so I think that is reflected in our work. We tolerate demanding patients a bit more. Some Americans tell us, how can you tolerate that patient? I would have told him off a long time ago.

In summary, the theme of an obligation to care reflected the Phillipine-American nurses' strong belief that bedside nursing is truly the core of nursing. This value conflicted with the attitude of some American nurses that the physical care of clients is devalued work with low prestige, and should therefore be delegated to ancillary personnel.

Differences in Locus of Control. *Locus of control* refers to the degree of control that individuals feel that they have over events. People who feel in control of their environment have an **internal locus of control**. People who believe that luck, fate, or chance control their lives have an **external locus of control**.

Health care professionals who are trained in the United States typically have an internal locus of control. American physicians and health care professionals feel that it is their duty to diagnose disorders, plan interventions, carry out procedures, and do everything possible to save the client's life.

Conversely, health care professionals from cultures that promote an external locus of control (some Mexican-Americans, Appalachians, and Puerto Ricans) may have a more fatalistic attitude toward their clients, and thus feel that they cannot control matters of life and death. For example, when a client who is expected to die does die on the operating room table, care providers with an external locus of control may be puzzled when the hospital administration asks for a quality review of the case (Giger & Davidhizar, 1996).

Finally, the cultural beliefs of some American Indians, Chinese-Americans, and Japanese-Americans may not fall under the concept of locus of control. These cultural groups believe themselves to be in harmony with nature, rather than being controlled by nature, or in control of nature (Giger & Davidhizar, 1996).

Differences in Time Orientation

Recall from Chapter 2 that cultural groups are either past- present- or future-oriented. Americans generally value the future over the present. Southern blacks and Puerto Ricans value the present over the future. Southern Appalachians, traditional Chinese-Americans, and Mexican-Americans value the present.

The ways in which different cultural groups value time can create challenges in the health care workplace. For example, people who work in the operating room (OR) must be both future and present oriented. To plan and adhere to the OR schedule, the person must be future oriented, and abide by the calendar and clock. However, once the surgical procedure begins, the surgeon and other health care professionals must now switch to a present orientation (Giger & Davidhizar, 1996).

Staff meetings also are influenced by the time orientation of staff members. For instance, staff members who are meeting to plan for the future, may become annoyed with members who want to spend all of the time on present-day problems and issues.

Educational Differences

The fact that foreign health care professionals are educated differently than American health care professionals raises yet another potential barrier to communication. Health care education outside of the United States is less theory-oriented, focusing primarily on the development of clinical skills. Also there is less emphasis on meeting the psychosocial needs of clients. As a result, foreign-educated health care professionals may be less inclined to use therapeutic touch with clients, or to engage clients in conversations that build trust and rapport.

Also, because most non-Western cultures value emotional restraint, foreign-educated health care professionals may not be trained to intervene when clients are experiencing grief or loss. Moreover, health care professionals from non-Western cultures may feel that grief and loss are private family matters, and that it is the family's responsibility to assist the client (Burner, 1990).

Another cultural difference in the education of health care professionals revolves around *who* provides the majority of care—the health care professionals, the family, or the client. Recall that the Philippine-American health care professionals felt it was *their duty* to give clients complete physical care. Other health care professionals, educated outside of the United States, may have been taught that it is the *family's duty* to bathe the client and provide personal care. For example, in the far East and in rural hospitals in Africa, a family member usually bathes the client. As a result of this training, a foreign-born professional may be reluctant to provide morning care to clients.

In contrast, health care professionals educated in the United States are taught that clients should perform *self-care* whenever possible. In keeping with the American values of independence and self-reliance, American health care professionals encourage clients to be ambulatory, active, and self-sufficient as soon as possible.

Even when health care professionals are from other English-speaking countries, they are educated differently than American health care professionals. English professionals, taught under the system of socialized medicine, may find it difficult to adjust to the concept that health care in the United States is a business, and physicians are in private practice. These health care professionals may not be familiar with physician referral services, charging clients for supplies, or the use of extreme measures to prolong the lives of terminally ill clients.

Language Differences

Language differences, perhaps more than any other barrier, raise the potential for serious miscommunications between health care professionals. Today, large medical centers in the United States may be primarily staffed by health care professionals and physicians for whom English is a second language. For example, in urban medical centers on the East Coast, it is not unusual to hear Filipino health care professionals and Haitian health care professionals attempting to communicate with a resident physician who has been educated in India. Unless these care givers take the time to clarify their communications, serious errors may result. Even when only one individual is foreign born, the potential for miscommunication still exists (especially over the telephone), unless words are clarified by a co-worker or physician.

> **Example:** A Filipino licensed practical nurse who was temporarily assigned to an unfamiliar medical unit transcribed a telephone order from a physician. The physician said: "Give Johnson 50 ml of Demerol for pain. If she is still complaining of pain after an hour, call me and I'll increase the dosage." When transcribing the order, the medical assistant missed the physician's reference to the client as *she,* a common error among Filipinos and some Chinese and Japanese speakers. Mr. Johnson, who happened to be on the same ward, might have received the medication, had another licensed practical nurse not questioned the order.

Language differences can also create communication problems between clients and health care professionals. Clients may feel apprehensive when they are assigned a foreign professional (Burner, 1990). Clients may complain that foreign health care professionals do not understand what they are saying. For instance, the health care professional may not comprehend the client's request for a pain medication or assistance.

Furthermore, nonverbal communication can create misunderstandings. For example, an Asian health care professional may think that it is rude to sustain prolonged eye contact with a client; the client, on the other hand, may interpret the lack of eye contact as disinterest. As a result of this confusion, the client may request an American health care professional, which in turn, could cause the foreign health care professional to feel inadequate and disrespected.

Language differences are also a source of friction between American and foreign health care professionals. When frictions escalate, foreign health care professionals form cliques in a clinic. By speaking in their native language and excluding English-speaking professionals, foreign health care professionals may feel unified, even though they are alienating themselves even further from the rest of the health care staff (Burner, 1990). English-speaking health care professionals may believe that they are being talked about by the foreign professionals, and thus demand that personnel speak only English on the unit. Foreign health care professionals, denied the right to speak their own language at work, can feel even more threatened and angry, which erects further obstacles to transcultural communication.

BRIDGES TO TRANSCULTURAL COMMUNICATION BETWEEN HEALTH CARE PROFESSIONALS

Although there are many barriers to transcultural communication between health care professionals, there are also numerous ways to bridge the gap that separates people from different cultures. This section presents techniques for communicating with team members who have different cultural backgrounds, and who may not speak fluent English. We will also explore the important role of the health care manager in promoting transcultural communication and resolving workplace conflicts.

Using Transcultural Communication to Work With Team Members

Health care professionals have a responsibility to communicate clearly with each other, with physicians, with other health care professionals, and with unlicensed assistive personnel. Murky communications can result in errors that compromise client care. Thus, health care professionals must make every effort to communicate clearly.

If you are assigned to work with health care professionals who are from a different culture, and who speak English as a second language, try these techniques to facilitate communication:

- Recognize that your co-worker probably has an educational background in health care that is very different from your own.

- Acknowledge that the co-worker's value system and perception of what constitutes "good client care" may differ from your own.

- Try to assess your co-worker's level of understanding of verbal and written communication. For example, ask a co-worker to explain a physician's order to you in her own words. It also helps to assess a client with the co-worker, and note what terms the person uses to describe the client's signs and symptoms.

- In communicating with health care professionals for whom English is a second language, avoid the use of slang terms and regional expressions. For example, Chinese, Japanese, and Filipino health care professionals may not understand such terms as *piggybacking, doing a double,* or *rigging something to work.*

- Do provide your co-worker with resources such as written procedures and protocols that may help to reinforce your verbal communication.

- Remember to praise your co-worker's competency in technical skills. Inspiring self-confidence in foreign health care professionals will make it easier for them to ask for assistance when needed.

- Appreciate the knowledge that you can gain by working alongside skilled health care professionals from another culture. Observe how foreign health care professionals relate to clients who are from their culture. If you have an open mind, working with foreign co-workers can increase your knowledge of other cultures, enrich your work in health care, and foster personal growth (Tilki, 1994).

- When offering constructive criticism, try to use *I statements* instead of *you statements.* For example: "I think that it's very important to address the client's emotional state when you chart" is better than saying "You never seem to chart anything about the client's emotional state."

- If you feel you cannot achieve effective communication with a co-worker, request to work with another person. You do not want to be held accountable for the actions of health care professionals with whom you cannot communicate.

- Report to your supervisor if you feel that a health care professional or a physician is endangering clients due to language difficulties or different cultural values. Record any problems that occur, and keep a copy of the notes you provide to your supervisor.

Sometimes you may need to work with a foreign physician who is difficult to understand due to language differences or a strong accent. In this case, do not take verbal orders, particularly over the telephone. Even when an order is written, take the time to clarify the order with the physician. As clients may also find it difficult to understand a foreign physician, you will need to listen carefully, and then explain the physician's remarks to the client.

Another group of health care workers who may have difficulty understanding and speaking English are unlicensed assistive personnel (Walton & Waszkiewiez, 1997). If you are called upon to supervise an unlicensed worker who speaks English as a second language, follow these cautions:

- Delegate appropriate tasks to an unlicensed worker. Match assignments to the worker's level of understanding and skill.

- Do not stop at just delegating an assignment or giving instructions. Instead, make sure that the worker understands your instructions.

- Restate your instructions in clear, concrete terms, and give a demonstration of a procedure if necessary.

- To reduce miscommunication, check for understanding by asking the worker to repeat instructions or do a return demonstration.

- If you are still not satisfied that the communication between the two of you is accurate and effective, repeat your directions again and request a repeat demonstration.

- Establish a time frame for the worker to complete assigned tasks. For example, "I want you to feed Mr. Brown before you get Mr. Black out of bed."

- Observe how the worker communicates with clients and performs duties.

- Give workers clear feedback concerning their communication skills and performance of duties. If the worker has performed a procedure incorrectly, offer suggestions for improvement. Demonstrate the procedure as it should be done, and ask for a return demonstration.

- If, in spite of your best efforts, the worker is still unable to perform due to language difficulties, ask your supervisor to work with the person. Again, you do not want to be held responsible for a worker with whom you cannot communicate.

Using Transcultural Communication to Manage a Diverse Staff

To effectively manage a multicultural work force, a health care manager must possess the same high level of cultural sensitivity that is required to successfully care for clients from other cultures. Health care managers face many complex issues as they go about their role of supervising health care professionals and assistive personnel from around the world. The three major issues encountered by health care professionals in administrative positions are:

1. clashes in values that arise between foreign health care professionals and professionals trained in the United States

2. language differences that disrupt hospital communications

3. tensions and conflicts between staff members that are frequently rooted in racial and cultural differences, and which can escalate into lawsuits.

Major tasks of the health care manager in a diverse hospital environment include:

1. helping American health care professionals acknowledge that professionals from other cultures have values and ideas that are as valuable as their own

2. establishing opportunities for improving transcultural communication between staff members

3. resolving conflicts between staff members

4. resolving tensions between clients and foreign health care professionals

5. helping foreign nurses acclimate to American ways.

Improving Transcultural Communication Between Staff Members. To actively manage a diverse health care staff, Jamieson and O'Mara (1991) have laid out a broad, six-step program for health care managers to follow:

1. determine which cultural groups are represented on staff

2. understand the organization's values and goals

3. decide on what is best for the future of the organization

4. analyze present conditions within the organization

5. plan ways to reach the desired future state, and decide how to manage transitions

6. evaluate the results.

More specifically, health care managers might consider using the following approaches to diminish tensions between staff members and improve transcultural communication:

- Plan informal meetings for health care professionals to discuss their cultural values. For example, it may benefit Asian health care professionals to share their cultural values concerning respect for authority with American-born health care professionals.

- Provide cultural workshops, and ask knowledgeable individuals to present information about the values, behaviors, and communication patterns of the different cultural groups that are represented on staff.

- Provide classes in English as a second language for foreign health care professionals who do not speak fluent English, or who have difficulty pronouncing words.

- Establish a program for orienting foreign health care professionals to the clinic hospital or agency (Jein & Harris, 1989). The orientation program should be designed to help newcomers adjust to the new work environment. It is helpful to assign new health care professionals to a preceptor who will assist in the orientation process. If possible, the preceptor should be a member of the health care professional's cultural group. For maximum benefits, the health care manager needs to interview new health care professionals every week to find out how that person is adapting to the new medical culture (Burner, 1996; Williams & Rodgers, 1993).

- Plan potluck events where health care professionals and other staff members can socialize and discuss cultural differences informally, in a relaxed environment. For example, each unit in the hospital might plan one potluck event per shift on a monthly basis. Potluck meals could be planned around a cultural theme; for instance a traditional Vietnamese dinner one month, and a traditional Costa Rican meal the next month (Burner, 1990).

- Confer with specialists in transcultural communication; also hire experts to identify potential areas of conflict, and resolve conflicts peacefully before they erupt into legal battles.

Using Transcultural Communication to Resolve Workplace Conflicts. Despite a health care manager's best efforts, serious conflicts may still arise between staff members who are from different races and cultures. Conflicts develop in a diverse work environment because people from different cultures are likely to perceive situations differently, and thus react to situations in ways that reflect their cultural values. Depending on their culture, people may react to a conflict with anger, denial, silence, distrust, annoyance, or resignation.

Styles of **conflict resolution** are also based in culture. Mainstream American culture emphasizes standing up for your rights, assertiveness, confrontation, and litigation. Traditional Asian cultures and some Native American cultures promote cooperation with others, and the avoidance of interpersonal conflicts. Arabs use mediation to settle conflicts and disputes. Mediation helps all parties come to a reasonable compromise while allowing everyone to save face (Jein & Harris, 1989). Because resolutions to conflict differ, health care managers must become experts in assessing conflict situations, and consciously deciding on the appropriate resolution style (Lowenstein & Glanville, 1995).

In a study of racial and status conflict among nurse administrators, staff nurses, and nursing assistants, the researchers found that employment disputes go through a process before they erupt into a legal dispute (Lowenstein & Glanville, 1995; Felstiner, 1981). During this process, an **unperceived injurious experience** (unPIE) is transformed into a **perceived injurious experience** (PIE). The steps of this transformation are as follows:

1. *Naming:* At this stage, a person or group recognizes that a particular experience has been injurious. An unPIE is transformed into a PIE.

2. *Blaming:* The PIE is transformed into a grievance, and the injured party blames another person, group, or social entity for the injury.

3. *Claiming:* The injured party now confronts the accused party or social entity, and demands remedial action.

4. Once a claim has been made, the claim is either rejected by the institution, or it is resolved with both sides coming to an agreement, or it advances into a lawsuit.

Researchers noted that the transformation of unPIEs into PIEs depends on (1) the organizational hierarchy that establishes the norms of expected behavior, and also the methods for resolving grievances, and (2) the particular characteristics of the individuals who are involved in the legal or labor dispute. Individual characteristics include each person's age, experience, socioeconomic status, personality type, degree of job satisfaction, social position, commitment to cultural values, and perception of prejudice within the organization.

COMMUNICATION CONSIDERATIONS

A knowledgeable health care manager can do much to help prevent the transformation of unPIEs into PIEs, and the escalation of conflicts into legal disputes. The more health care managers understand about the cultures represented in their institution, the better able they will be to resolve conflicts quickly.

Ellis and Hartley (1995) suggest eight steps that a health care manager can take to resolve conflicts within a group. The health care manager should:

1. Conduct a thorough self-assessment. Managers must ask themselves if they really understand the situation that is at the root of the conflict, and if they have any biases or prejudices against the people involved.

2. Analyze the issues or conditions that have created the conflict.

3. Review the analysis, adjust negative attitudes, and try to eliminate any biases that might interfere with solving the problem.

4. Schedule a meeting for all of the people who are involved in the conflict. The manager needs to notify the participants well in advance of the meeting, so they start thinking about solutions.

5. Encourage people at the meeting to speak openly about their feelings and viewpoints. Take every suggestion for solving the problem seriously.

6. Summarize all of the solutions that group members have suggested.

7. Help the group narrow the choices for action down to the one or two interventions that appear to be the best.

8. Put together a plan for implementing the choices for action. Following the meeting, the manager should send everyone a *written plan of action* and a *time line* that is based on the group's decisions.

Not all conflicts can be resolved in informal group meetings. In a serious legal or labor dispute, the hospital or agency may need to call in experts to negotiate, mediate, or arbitrate a settlement. Negotiation, mediation, and arbitration are *alternative dispute resolution remedies* that organizations use to avoid lengthy, costly, and stressful court hearings (Aiken, 1994; Lowenstein & Glanville, 1995).

- **Negotiation** involves compromising or coming to terms about a specific matter; for example, the terms of a contract. Negotiators help the involved parties solve conflicts by reaching a compromise, in which each party gives in on some points in order to gain certain advantages.

- **Mediation** involves the use of mediators who are neutral third parties. Mediators help both sides of a conflict identify their needs and come to an agreement.

- **Arbitration** is frequently used to resolve major employer–employee conflicts. The involved parties select a neutral third-party arbitrator who is an expert in the area of contention. The arbitrator hears the case and renders a decision.

Reducing Tensions Between Foreign Health Care Professionals and Clients.

In addition to resolving conflicts between staff members, health care managers sometimes need to reduce tensions between clients and foreign professionals. Health care professionals in administrative positions may face complaints from white clients who are being cared for by health care professionals who are not native English speakers.

For example, a Filipino health care professional whose primary language is Tagalog, may place the accent on the second syllable of each word, which is a characteristic speech pattern. The supervisor may need to assure clients that this Filipino health care professional is clinically competent, despite the pronunciation of English.

The health care manager may also request that health care professionals speak only English in all public areas of the hospital or agency. The point is that clients may become nervous when they hear health care professionals speaking a foreign language in their immediate environment. Clients may wonder if their foreign health care professional will understand them and provide for their needs (Burner, 1990).

Finally, health care managers may want to help some foreign health care professionals with their nonverbal communication. For example, the health care manager could encourage some foreign health care professionals to increase eye contact with their clients. The manager should explain that such instructions or suggestions are not intended to alter the foreign health care professional's culture, but rather to improve the individual's transcultural communication with American clients and health care professionals.

TESTING YOUR KNOWLEDGE

Circle the correct answer.

1. Select the fastest growing health care occupational group.
   a. registered nurses
   b. pharmacists
   c. unlicensed ancillary personnel
   d. physician assistants

2. Health care professionals with an internal locus of control
   a. have usually been educated outside of the United States.
   b. believe that it is impossible to control matters of life and death.
   c. believe care providers should do everything to save a person's life.
   d. believe that their lives depend on fate or luck.

3. In a study of Philippine-American nurses, the theme of *obligation to care* was expressed by
   a. dedication to work and a strong sense of duty.
   b. primary attention to the client's physical needs.
   c. an obligation to respect physicians and follow their orders.
   d. all of the above

4. Select the action you should take if you are working with health care professionals who are not providing safe client care due to language or cultural difference.
   a. Confront the person about the problem.
   b. Try to prevent a serious conflict by ignoring the problem.
   c. Talk with co-workers about the problem.
   d. Provide your supervisor with a written report of dates and incidents.

5. When a neutral third party hears a case and renders a decision, the process is called
   a. negotiation.
   b. mediation.
   c. arbitration.
   d. due process.

UNIT FIVE
EVALUATION

EVALUATING YOUR TRANSCULTURAL COMMUNICATION SKILLS WITH OTHER HEALTH CARE PROFESSIONALS

The following exercises will highlight some of the concepts that we discussed in Chapter 13, and they will also help you to evaluate the progress that you have made in your interactions with care professionals from other cultures.

Exercise One: Evaluating Your Personal Objectives

When you began to study this Unit, you were asked to select and write down your personal objectives for learning these new materials. Please review those objectives now.

1. To what extent have you met each objective that you selected from the list of objectives? _____

_____

_____

2. To what extent have you met the personal objectives that you listed?

_____

_____

_____

3. Have you developed any new objectives since you started this Unit?

_____

_____

_____

_____

Exercise Two: Evaluating Your Personal Responses to Working With Care Professionals From Different Cultures

Now that you have studied this Unit, and you are more aware of your daily interactions with health care professionals from other cultures, redo Exercise Two from the self-assessment section of this Unit. Select the answer that best describes your point of view *now* that you have completed the Unit, and spent some time recording transcultural interactions in your diary.

279

	Agree	Neutral	Disagree
I would rather work with American health care professionals than foreign health care professionals.	_____	_____	_____
I find it frustrating to work with health care professionals or physicians who are not proficient in English.	_____	_____	_____
If I thought that a health care professional or physician was not fulfilling duties due to cultural or language problems, I would hesitate to report them for fear that I would be considered prejudiced.	_____	_____	_____
I enjoy working with skilled foreign health care professionals. I feel that I can learn a lot from them.	_____	_____	_____
I like to attend classes and informal meetings where I can learn more about how health care professionals from other countries are educated.	_____	_____	_____
I do not feel prepared to work with or supervise an unlicensed assistive worker who has some problems with understanding English.	_____	_____	_____

Exercise Three: Reviewing *Your Transcultural Interaction Diary*

1. Have you had any *positive interactions* with health care professionals from other cultures? _____

_____

What communication skills did you use that helped to make the interaction a positive one? _____

_____

Is there anything that you could have done that would have improved your interaction even more? _____

_____

2. Have you had any *difficult or unsuccessful interactions* with health care professionals from other cultures?_____

What caused the interaction to be difficult or to fail in its intent?

_____

What could you have done to prevent the problem?

_____

Exercise Four: Evaluating Your Readiness For Communicating With Health Care Professionals From Other Cultures

Write a brief response to these questions, which are drawn from topics discussed in Chapter 13.

1. List three different ways in which language differences can create problems in the workplace.

   a. _____

   b. _____

   c. _____

2. Discuss the attributes of health care that prevent health care professionals from openly confronting racism in their profession.

   a. _____

   b. _____

   c. _____

3. When working with a foreign co-worker, what can you do to assess the worker's level of understanding of verbal and written English?

   _____

   _____

   _____

4. Describe at least five techniques that you can use to facilitate communication with a health care professional from a foreign country or different culture?

   a. _____

   b. _____

   c. _____

   d. _____

   e. _____

5. What should you do when a foreign physician who is difficult to understand asks you to take a verbal order? _____

   _____

   _____

6. What cautions should you observe when supervising an unlicensed worker who speaks limited English?

a. _____

b. _____

c. _____

d. _____

e. _____

f. _____

7. What are the four stages during which an unperceived injurious experience (unPIE) is transformed into a perceived injurious experience (PIE)?

a. _____

b. _____

c. _____

d. _____

8. How can conflicts between staff members be resolved without having to resort to a lawsuit?

_____

_____

_____

_____

_____

_____

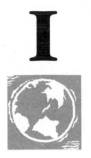

ORGANIZATIONS AND AGENCIES

Because this information is of a time sensitive nature, and URL addresses may change or be deleted, you are encouraged to also conduct your searches by association and/or topic.

PROFESSIONAL ORGANIZATIONS

American Anthropological Association
Society For Linguistic Anthropology (SLA)
Society For Medical Anthropology (SMA)
4350 N. Fairfax Drive, Suite 640
Arlington, VA 22203-1620
Phone: 703-528-1902
Fax: 703-528-3546
www.ameranthassn.org

American Association of Medical Assistants
20 North Wacker Drive
Suite 1575
Chicago, IL 60606-2903
Phone: 800-228-2262

American Association for Medical Transcription
PO Box 576187
Modesto, CA 95357-6187
Phone: 800-982-2182
FAX: 209-551-9317
www.aamt.org

American College of Radiography
1891 Preston White Drive
Preston, VA 20191
Phone: 800-227-5463
www.acr.org

American Dental Assistants Association
203 North LaSalle Street
Suite 1320
Chicago, IL 60601-1225
Phone: 312-541-1550
FAX: 312-541-1496

American Dental Association
211 East Chicago Avenue
Chicago, IL 60611
Phone: 800-621-8099
www.ada.org

American Dental Hygienist Association
444 North Michigan Avenue
Suite 3400
Chicago, IL 60611
Phone: 312-440-8900
www.adha.org

American Health Information Management Association
919 North Michigan Avenue
Suite 1400
Chicago, IL 60611-1683
Phone: 312-787-2672
www.ahima.org

American Medical Technologists
710 Higgins Road
Park Ridge, IL 60068
Phone: 800-275-1268

American Nurses' Association
600 Maryland Avenue, S.W.
Suite 100 West
Washington. DC 20024
Phone: 800-274-4ANA *or*
202-651-7000
Fax: 202-651-7001
www.ana.org

American Physical Therapy Association
1111 North Fairfax Street
Alexandria, VA 22314
Phone: 703-684-2782
www.apta.org

American Registry of Radiologic Technologists
1255 Northland Drive
St. Paul, MN 55120-1155
Phone: 651-687-0048
www.arrt.org

Asian-Pacific Islander Nurses Association
252 Sileck Street
Clifton, NJ 07013
Phone: 973-279-8473

Canadian Nurses Association
50 The Driveway
Ottawa, Ontario K2P 1E2
Phone: 800-361-8404 *or* 613-237-2133
Fax: 613-237-3520
www.can-nurses.ca

Council on Nursing and Anthropology
Nursing Department
Southeast Missouri State University
Cape Girardeau, MO 63701

International Association of Administrative Professionals
10502 NW Ambassador Drive
PO Box 20404
Kansas City, MO 64195-0404
Phone: 816-891-6600
www.iap-hg.org

National Association of Dental Laboratories
8201 Greensboro Drive
Suite 300
McLean, VA 22102
Phone: 703-610-9035
http://www.nadl.org

National Association of Hispanic Nurses
1501 16th Street, NW
Washington, DC 20036
Phone: 202-387-5000
Fax: 202-797-4353

National Black Nurses Association, Inc.
1511 K Street NW, Suite 415
Washington, DC 20005
Phone: 202-393-6870
Fax: 202-347-3808

National Council for International Health (NCIH)
1701 K Street, NW, Suite 600
Washington, DC 20006
Phone: 202-833-5900
Fax: 202-833-0075
www.ncih.org

Native American Nurses Association
927 Treadale Lane
Cloquet, MN 55720

Philippine Nurses Association of America, Inc.
489 Morris Avenue
Boonton, NJ 07005

Society of Medical Interpreters (SOMI)
c/o Cross Cultural Health Care Program
Pacific Medical Center
1200 12th Avenue S.
Seattle, WA 98144 *or*
P.O. Box 3304
Seattle, WA 98144
Phone: 206-621-4053
Fax: 206-326-2408

Transcultural Nursing Society
c/o Madonna University College of
    Nursing and Health
36600 Schoolcraft Road
Livonia, MI 48150-1173
Phone: 888-432-5470
Fax: 313-432-5463

GOVERNMENT AGENCIES

Office of Alternative Medicine (OAM/NIH)
National Institutes of Health
OAM Clearinghouse
P.O. Box 8218
Silver Spring, MD 20907-8218
Phone: 888-644-6226
Fax: 301-495-4957
www.altmed.od.nih.gov/oam/

Office of Minority Health Resource Center
8403 Colesville Road
Suite 910
Silver Spring, MD 20910
Phone: 800-444-6472
www.omhrc.gov

U.S. Department of Commerce, Economics and Statistics Administration
Bureau of the Census
Herbert C. Hoover Building
14th Street and Constitution Avenue
    NW
Washington, DC 20230
Phone: 202-482-2000
www.census.gov *or* www.doc.gov

U.S. Department of Health and Human Services
U.S. Public Health Service
Indian Health Service, IHS
Parklawn Building
5600 Fishers Lane
Rockville, MD 20857
Phone: 301-443-3593
Fax: 301-443-0507
www.tuscon.his.gov

U.S. Department of Health and Human Services
U.S. Public Health Service
Office of Minority Health, OMH
Rockwall II Building, Suite 1000
5600 Fishers Lane
Rockville, MD 20857
Phone: 800-444-6472 *or*
    301-443-5224
Fax: 301-443-8280
www.hhs.gov

ETHNIC AND MINORITY ORGANIZATIONS AND AGENCIES

American-Arab Antidiscrimination Committee (ABD)
4201 Connecticut Avenue NW
Suite 300
Washington, DC 20008
Phone: 202-244-2990
Fax: 202-244-3196
www.adc.org

American-Arab Relations Committee (AARC)
Box 416
New York, NY 10017
Phone: 516-889-0005

American Civil Liberties Union (ACLU)
1215 Broad Street, 18th Floor
New York, NY 10004-2400
www.aclu.org

American Indian Culture Research Center (AICRC)
P.O. Box 98, Blue Cloud Abbey
Marvin, SD 57251-0098
Phone: 605-432-5528
Fax: 605-432-4754
www.bluecloud.org

American Indian Heritage Foundation
6051 Arlington Blvd.
Falls Church, VA 22044
Phone: 202-463-4267
Fax: 703-532-1921
www.indians.org

American Indian Institute
University of Oklahoma
555 Constitution Avenue, Suite 237
Norman, OK 73072-7820
Phone: 405-325-4127
Fax: 405-325-7757

American Jewish Committee
Jacob Blaustein Building
165 E. 56th Street
New York, NY 10022
Phone: 212-751-4000
Fax: 212-838-2120
www.ajc.org

Anti-Defamation League (Seeks to stop defamation of Jewish people)
823 United Nations Plaza
New York, NY 10017
Phone: 212-490-2525
Fax: 212-867-0779

Asia Society
725 Park Avenue
New York, NY 10021
Phone: 212-288-6400
Fax: 212-517-8315

Asian American Legal Defense and Education Fund (AALDEF)
99 Hudson Street, 12th Floor
New York, NY 10013
Phone: 212-966-5932
Fax: 212-966-4303

Cultural Integration Fellowship (CIF)
360 Cumberland Street
San Francisco, CA 94114-2516
Phone: 415-626-2442 *or*
2650 Fulton Street
San Francisco, CA 94118-4026
Phone: 415-386-9590

Islamic Information Center of America (IICA)
830 E. Old Willow Road
Prospect Heights, IL 60070
Phone: 847-541-8141
Fax: 847-824-8436

Islamic Information Office
1935 D. Aleo Place
Honolulu, HI 96822
www.iio.org

National Association for the Advancement of Colored People (NAACP)
4805 Mt. Hope Dr.
Baltimore, MD 21215
Phone: 410-486-9147
Fax: 410-764-7357
NAACP Information Hotline:
   410-521-4939
or
Washington Bureau
1025 Vermont Avenue, NW, Suite 1120
Washington, DC 20005
Phone: 202-638-2269
www. naacp.org

National Latina Health Organization (NLHO)
P.O. Box 7567
Oakland, CA 94601
Phone: 510-534-1362
Fax: 510-534-1364

National Urban League (NUL)
120 Wall Street
New York, NY 10005
Phone: 212-558-5300
Fax: 212-558-5332
www.nul.org

INTERNATIONAL AGENCIES

International Council of Nurses (ICN)
3, place Jean Marteau
1201 Geneva, Switzerland
Fax: 41-22-9080101
Phone: 41-22-9080100

National Council for International Health (NCIH)
1701 K Street, NW, Suite 600
Washington, DC 20006
Phone: 202-833-5900
Fax: 202-833-0075
www.ncih.org

Pan American Health Organization
Nursing Section, Health Services
   Division
525 23rd Street, NW
Washington, DC 20037
Phone: 202-974-3000
Fax: 202-338-3663
www.paho.org

Project HOPE
The People to People Health
   Foundation, Inc.
Health Sciences Education Center,
   Carter Hall
Milkwood, VA 22646
Phone: 800-544-4673 *or*
   540-837-2100
Fax: 540-837-1813
www.projhope.org

World Health Organization (WHO)
Headquarters:
Avenue Appia 20
1211 Geneva 27
Switzerland
Phone: 41 22 791 21 11
Regional Office **(WHO)**:
525 23rd Street NW
Washington, DC 20037-2832
Phone: 202-974-3000
Fax: 202-974-3663
www.who.org

REFUGEE CENTERS AND PROGRAMS

Central American Refugee Center (CARECEN)
3112 Mount Pleasant Street NW
Washington, DC 20010
Phone: 202-328-9799
Fax: 202-328-2300
or
91 N. Franklin Street
Hempstead, NY 11550
Phone: 516-489-8330

Haitian Refugee Center (HRC)
119 NE 54th Street
Miami, FL 33137
Phone: 305-757-8538
Fax: 305-758-2444

Refugee Policy Group (RPG)
1424 16th Street NW, Suite 401
Washington, DC 20036-2211
Phone: 202-387-3015
Fax: 202-667-5034

United States Committee for Refugees (USCR)
1717 Massachusetts Avenue NW, Suite 701
Washington, DC 20036
Phone: 202-347-3507
Fax: 202-347-3418
www.irsa-uscr.org

TELEPHONE INFORMATION LINES

Centers for Disease Control
Immunizations and Vaccinations
Information Hotline
800-232-2522
www.cdc.gov

Immigration and Naturalization Service (INS)
Toll free request phone number for INS forms:
800-870-FORM (3676)
www.ins.usdoj.gov

II

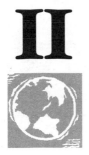

ANNOTATED LIST OF SUGGESTED BOOKS AND FILMS WITH A TRANSCULTURAL THEME

FICTION

A Lesson Before Dying by Ernest Gaines (1993) is set in rural Louisiana in 1948. This is the story of a young black man who is falsely accused by the white community, and who finds dignity as he faces the electric chair for a robbery and murder which he did not commit. In this and other novels, Gaines stresses the need for black men to "stand tall" and face injustice and adversity with courage.

A Treasury of African-American Christmas Stories compiled and edited by Bettye Collier-Thomas (1997), studies black culture at the beginning of the 20th century through short stories, poetry, and newspaper and magazine stories. This anthology also provides short biographies of the authors, describing each author's contribution to black literature, black culture, and American society.

Blu's Hanging by Ann Yamanaka (1997), a drama set in the author's native Hawaii, depicts the harrowing lives of three destitute children who are left to survive on the Island of Molokai following their mother's death. Yamanaka, a Japanese-American writer, has won awards for her lyrical poems and realistic novels about Hawaiian life.

Breath, Eyes, Memory by Edwidge Danticat (1994) is the story of Sophie, a young girl who grows up in Haiti, spends a rebellious adolescence in New York, and then returns to Haiti to reconcile with her mother. This powerful debut novel by Haitian author Danticat has been compared with the early novels of black Nobel Laureate, Toni Morrison.

Dark Blue Suit And Other Stories by Peter Bacho (1997) contains a dozen semi-autobiographical stories that take place in the Filipino community of Seattle, Washington. Several of the stories describe Bacho's pursuit of the art of boxing at the "Bruce Lee school" as a way for him to gain respect—"the most precious currency of the poor and colored."

Eating Chinese Food Naked by Mei Ng (1998) is a coming-of-age story about Ruby Lee, a Chinese, Columbia University graduate who returns home to her parents who work and live in a laundry in Queens, New York. The novel explores the problems that Ruby experiences as she tries to reconcile contemporary American ways with the traditional cultural values of her parents.

Fragile Night by Stella Pope Duarte (1997) is a collection of 15 short slice-of-life stories about life in the barrio. Her stories describe the lives of long-suffering Latina women, who in the Latino cultural tradition, feel that they must put up with their husbands' infidelities and abuse.

Go Tell It On The Mountain by James Baldwin (1953), a first novel, was the largely autobiographical work that established Baldwin as a writer. In addition to his essays, Baldwin wrote other influential novels including *Giovanni's Room, Another Country,* and *Tell Me How Long The Train's Been Gone.* Baldwin was deeply involved in the civil rights movement, and his writings focused on the racism that blacks face in America.

Honey, Hush!: An Anthology of African American Women's Humor edited by Daryl Cumber Dance (1997), covers 200 years of black women's biting humor and satire that ranges from slave narratives to contemporary fiction by Terry McMillan, author of *Waiting To Exhale* and *How Stella Got Her Groove Back.*

In Broken WigWag by Suchi Asano (1997) tells the story of Satomi, a Japanese expatriate who has been living for 8 years in a cramped apartment in lower Manhattan. Satomi longs for a more fulfilling life but does not know where to find it. This novel provides an interesting look into the American Japanese community, and the everyday lives of young Japanese women.

Krik? Krak! by Edwidge Danticat (1996) is a collection of short fiction that depicts the difficulties and tragedies that are a part of everyday life in the author's war-torn homeland of Haiti. These stories also give the reader insight into the myths and folklore that has evolved through generations of Haitians.

Midnight Sandwiches And The Mariposa Express by Beatriz Rivera (1997) is a witty first novel that tells the story of Cuban immigrant Trish Izquierdo, who is a town councilwoman in a fictitious New Jersey town. The Mariposa Express is the town's popular cafeteria where Trish meets with other primarily Hispanic characters to discuss the latest town gossip and political scandals.

Night Talk by Elizabeth Cox (1997) opens during the racially turbulent 1950s, and depicts the growing friendship between two adolescent girls—one the daughter of a white Research biologist, and the other the daughter of a black domestic who works for the white family. The "night talks" between the girls who share a bedroom, and later their letters to each other, form a deeply personal basis for describing the drama of the civil rights movement.

Ourselves Among Others: Cross-Cultural Readings for Writers (3rd edition) by Carol J. Verburg (1994) is an anthology of cross-cultural short stories, memoirs, and essays by authors from all over the world. Among the authors are such highly regarded writers as Octavio Paz, Margaret Atwood, Günter Gass, Carlos Fuentes, and Simone de Beauvoir.

Paradise by Toni Morrison (1998), the author's seventh novel, takes place between the 1970s and late 1980s, and is set outside of the all-black town of Ruby, Oklahoma. The book describes the lives of a group of women who live in an old house called "The Convent." It also focuses on generational conflicts, racial conflicts, and the allusive meaning of paradise. The Nobel prize winning author has also written *The Bluest Eye, Song of Solomon,* and *Beloved* among other novels.

Short Fiction by Hispanic Writers of the United States edited by Nicolas Kanellos (1993) contains Puerto Rican, Cuban-American, and Mexican-American short fiction in which authors tell stories about Hispanic life in the United States.

Snow Falling On Cedars by David Guterson (1995) is a complex transcultural drama that on one level recounts the trial of Kubuo Miyamoto, a Japanese-American who is accused of murdering a local fisherman on San Piedro Island in Washington State. On a deeper level, the novel addresses the tragic fate of the Japanese residents of San Piedro Island who were sent into exile during World War II.

Sweetbitter: A Novel by Reginald Gibbons (1994) is a turn of the century tale set in East Texas. Gibbons tells the story of Reuben S. Sweetbitter, a young half-Choctaw, half white man who has lost contact with his Choctaw roots. The novel describes Sweetbitter's attempts to find his place in the world, his forbidden love relationship with a young white woman, and his flight with her to a place where they hope to find peace and acceptance.

The Joy Luck Club by Amy Tan (1989) is a collection of 16 interconnected stories that explore the complex transcultural relationships between four mothers who are Chinese immigrants born prior to World War II, and their four American-born daughters, who are first-generation Californians. *The Joyluck Club* was released as a motion picture in 1993.

The Lone Ranger And Tonto Fist Fight In Heaven by Sherman Alexie (1995) is a collection of short stories about Native Americans, which was used as the basis for *Smoke Signals*. This film, by and about young Native Americans, describes the journey of two young men from the reservation to Phoenix, Arizona to claim one of the father's ashes.

NONFICTION

A Country Of Strangers: Blacks and Whites In America by David K. Shipler (1997) is a record of the in-depth interviews of this former *New York Times* correspondent with hundreds of people across the United States. From his interviews, Shipler concluded that black Americans and white Americans have little knowledge or understanding of each other's lives.

Angela's Ashes by Frank McCourt (1996) is the gritty childhood memoir of the author's Irish childhood. McCourt describes how he grew up poor and miserable in the slums of Limerick, with a drunken father and a mother named Angela, who desperately tried to hold her starving family together.

Beyond The Godfather: Italian American Writers on the Real Italian American Experience edited by A. Kenneth Ciongoli and Jay Parini (1997) is a collection of 23 essays on Italian-American culture. The essays are divided into personal reflections on life as an Italian-American, the Italian-American literary tradition, and the Italian-American heritage.

Bloodlines: Odyssey of a Native Daughter by Janet Campbell (1998) contains the author's family history in seven autobiographical essays. Campbell is a member of the Coeur d'Alene tribe of northern Idaho.

Daughters of Kings: Growing Up as a Jewish Woman in America edited by Leslie Brody (1997), is a collection of academic essays written by 13 fellows of the Bunting Institute at Radcliffe College, which explores the topics of Jewish heritage and Jewish identity. Authors from many ethnic backgrounds describe their experiences either as Jewish women, or as non-Jewish women who are living and working in a Jewish community.

Death And Dying In Central Appalachia: Changing Attitudes and Practices by James K. Crissman (1994) uses photographs, archival sources, and interviews with over 400 mountain dwellers to explore the rituals associated with death, dying, and funeral customs in the Appalachian sections of Tennessee, Virginia, Kentucky, North Carolina, and West Virginia.

Double Burden: Black Women And Everyday Racism by Yanick St. Jean and Joe R. Feagin (1998), presents a study based on interviews and focus groups with 200 black women. In the book, the black women respondents describe their feelings of being "physically, morally, and spiritually stigmatized by a dominant culture."

Growing Up Chicana/o: An Anthology, edited by Tiffany Ana Lopez (1993) contains the writings of 20 authors. Each author describes the experience of being a child who grows up caught between rich Hispanic traditions and the need to assimilate into mainstream American culture.

Growing Up Native American: An Anthology, edited by Patricia Riley (1993) contains the essays and short stories of 22 authors whose writings span the years from the 19th century to the 1990s. Each of these authors explore the many challenges that are faced by Native American youths who are coming of age in the United States and Canada.

Heart of a Woman by Maya Angelou (1981) is the fourth volume of the acclaimed author's autobiography. In this book, Angelou looks back on her life as a Black woman in America, her civil rights work with Martin Luther King, and her fascinating encounters with such famous blacks as Billie Holiday and Malcolm X.

In Search of the Racial Frontier: African Americans in the American West by Quintard Taylor (1998) covers the era from the early 16th century to the present. The book documents how black Westerners struggled to integrate themselves into the larger society while working as doctors, lawyers, schoolteachers, newspaper editors, restaurant owners, barbershop owners, newspaper editors, waiters, and cooks.

James Baldwin: Collected Essays edited by Toni Morrison (1998) compiles Baldwin's influential essays that helped to expose the polarization of blacks and whites in America. This massive anthology contains several essay collections including *Notes of a Native Son* (1955), *Nobody Knows My Name* (1961), *The Fire Next Time* (1963), *No Name in the Street* (1972), *The Devil Finds Work* (1976), and a group of articles and interviews called *The Price of the Ticket* (1985) which was published two years before Baldwin's death from cancer.

Leaving Deep Water: The Lives of Asian American Women at the Crossroads of Two Cultures by Claire S. Chow (1998) presents Chow's study of racial identity; her interviews with 120 primarily middle-class, Asian-American women; and personal narrative. A psychotherapist, Chow learned that like herself, some of the women felt confused about their racial identity, while others were proud of their Asian heritage. Respondents who had grown up in racially integrated Hawaii had the fewest identity problems.

Makes Me Wanna Holler: A Young Black Man in America by Nathan McCall (1994) is a first-person account of a young black man who is from a decent family, but who is nevertheless lured into a life of crime and violence. At nineteen, McCall is sentenced to 12 years in prison for robbing a fast-food joint. In prison, McCall is exposed to books, then completes college while on parole, and then finally becomes a successful newspaper man on the *Washington Post.*

Miners And Medicine: West Virginia Memories by Claude A. Frazier, MD (1992) recalls Dr. Frazier's memories of the coal camps of Appalachia where his father was a camp doctor. The book describes the horrific health problems and hazardous, diseased working environment faced by the coal miners before the United Mine Workers of America promoted better working conditions and medical care.

Ono Ono Girl's Hula by Carolyn Lei-lanilau (1997) is a collection of humorous but angry short essays that address the problems inherent in being a person of mixed race in America. Lei-lanilau, a winner of the American Book Award for poetry, was raised in Hawaii by her Chinese mother and Hawaiian Turkish father before coming to the United States.

The Children by David Halberstam (1998) chronicles the lives of eight idealistic young black college students who evolved into leaders of the civil rights movement. The story covers five years, beginning with sit-ins in 1960 and ending with the passage of the Voting Rights Act of 1965.

The Famine Ships: The Irish Exodus to America by Edward Laxton (1998) is an illustrated chronicle of the experiences of the one million Irish immigrants who fled from their miserable lives in Ireland in the hope of finding peace and prosperity in America.

The Maria Paradox: How Latinas Can Merge Old World Traditions With New World Self-Esteem by Rosa Maria Gil and Carmen Inoa Vazquez (1996) asks this question: How can an Hispanic woman empower herself with North American ways, without giving up the valued Latin tradition that the female role is one of submission to male authority? To answer this question, the authors (both Latina psychotherapists) present Hispanic women with methods for balancing family and career demands, creating a sense of partnership within a traditional marriage, and standing up for their own feelings and rights.

The Nawal El Saadawi Reader: Selected Essays, 1970-1996 by Nawal el Saadawi (1997) is a collection of 23 essays written by a woman who is considered by some to be the leading authority on the status of women in the Arab world. Her essays cover a variety of topics ranging from women's health to the impact of Islamic fundamentalism on Arab women's movement toward political change.

The Rez Road Follies: Canoes, Casinos, Computers, and Birch Baskets by Jim Northrup (1997) humorously describes life on an Indian reservation and in a Federal boarding school for young Native Americans, as experienced by Northrup—a member of the Anishinaabe tribe, a newspaper columnist, and the author of *Walking the Rez Road*. With sadness and humor, Northrop recalls his days at the Federal school where he was taught about the ways of white society or, in his words, the "immigrant community."

Wisdom's Daughters: Conversations With Women Elders of Native America written and photographed by Steve Wall (1994) combines more than 100 photographs with the words of Native American women elders to paint a vivid portrait of a unified, harmonious philosophy of life.

With A Whoop And A Holler: A Bushel of Lore from Way Down South by Nancy Van Laan (1998) is a collection of fresh and funny Southern folklore, homespun tales, outlandish rhythms and riddles, old time superstitions, and ribald colloquialisms drawn from the bayous of Alabama, the mountains of Appalachia, and the intriguing culture of the deep South.

FILMS

Alamo Bay (1985) In a story that takes place in the late 1970s, Vietnamese refugees come to the Gulf Coast of Texas in hopes of building a new life in America. Instead, to their horror, the refugees come face to face with racist American fishermen and Ku Klux Klan members.

A ***Price Above Rubies*** (1998) An ultra-Orthodox Jewish (Hasidic) wife who lives in New York City, discovers that she can no longer play the traditional and sexually suppressed role expected of women in a patriarchal society. At first the unhappy wife looks for love with her brother-in-law who is a jeweler, but then finds sexual fulfillment with a Puerto Rican artist. The title *A Price Above Rubies* is drawn from a Biblical parable.

A ***Stranger Among Us*** (1992) In this transcultural police drama placed in Brooklyn, a policewoman goes to live in a close-knit Hasidic Jewish community where she searches for the "insider" who has murdered a community member. In the course of infiltrating this community, the brash, tough policewoman dons modest Hasidic female clothing, observes traditional dietary and religious customs, and even falls in love with a devout Hasidic scholar.

Driving Miss Daisy (1990) Based on a Pulitzer Prize winning play by Alfred Uhry, this film explores the unconventional, twenty-five year relationship between Miss Daisy—a strong-willed, Southern, Jewish widow, and her chauffeur Hoke Colburn—an illiterate, dignified, black widower. The film winds its way through many small adventures, little arguments, and reconciliations. In the end, when Miss Daisy is visited by Hoke in the nursing home, she finally realizes that despite their differences, her chauffeur is truly her best friend.

Falling Down (1993) A divorced white man who has lost his job as a defense worker, as well as the right to see his little daughter on her birthday, "cracks up" under the strain. Going on a rampage in East Los Angeles, this disenfranchised white male who feels violated and enraged, violently confronts a Korean grocery store owner, Mexican gang members, and a Neo Nazi. Finally he brings about his own death during a shoot-out with a police detective.

El Norte (1983) A Guatemalan brother and sister make a long and dangerous journey from their violence torn homeland to the United States, which they call *El Norte*. Once in Los Angeles, the young people, filled with hope, attempt to start new lives only to discover fresh obstacles and prejudices. One of the most unforgettable scenes in the film is when the sister is attacked and bitten by rats, as she and her brother fight their way across the border through subterranean tunnels.

Grand Avenue (Made for Cable, 1996) This slice-of-life made-for-television movie dramatizes the traumatic changes faced by a Native American mother and her children, who leave the reservation for a new life in an urban neighborhood. The family tries to start life over in a California town, only to be threatened by gangs and almost destroyed by neighborhood violence.

Heaven and Earth (1993) Preceded by *Platoon* (1986) and *Born On The Fourth of July* (1989), this is the third film in a trilogy about Vietnam by director Oliver Stone. The story follows the unhappy life of Le Ly, a young Vietnamese woman who marries an American Marine sergeant, and returns home with him to California. Unable to cope with her emotionally disturbed husband, Le Ly's life and marriage fall apart due to cultural clashes and post-war stress.

Lone Star (1996) Hispanics, blacks, and anglos attempt to live together in a Texas border town which was once dominated by a cruel, racist, and murderous white sheriff. This film dramatizes both the investigation of a 40-year-old murder mystery, and the love between the sheriff's son and the Mexican woman with whom he grew up.

Mi Familia (*My Family*, 1995) With a time frame that stretches from the 1920s to the present, *Mi Familia* traces the struggles of a Mexican-American family who call East Los Angeles home. A strong religious faith and a deep sense of togetherness help family members survive discrimination, racism, deportation, imprisonment, and the tragic death of a son.

Mississippi Masala (1992) This romantic comedy draws its title from its location (a small town in Mississippi) and masala, which is a blending of hot, multicolored, Indian spices. The story is about the transcultural love affair between Demetrius, a young black Mississippian and Mina, a young woman from Uganda, and the heat that their relationship generates in this traditional Southern community.

Mi Vita Loca (*My Crazy Life*, 1994) This offbeat, independent film explores life among the Latina girl gangs in Echo Park, a potentially violent ethnic area of Los Angeles. The writer/director Allison Anders, lived in this troubled neighborhood for several years, and spent time with the "homegirls" and their male friends. Her movie about *Sad Girl and Mousie* and the love they jealously share with a neighborhood drug dealer, gives the viewer a glimpse into the hopelessness of inner city life.

Mr. and Mrs. Loving (1996) A working class Southern couple, Mr. and Mrs. Loving, are driven out of their native state of Virginia because their mixed marriage violates antimiscegenation laws. A true story, the Lovings took their case to the Supreme Court, which abolished antimiscegenation laws in the early 1960s.

Not In This Town (1997) This is the true-life story of a Jewish family who stands up to a vicious Neo-Nazi clan in Billings Montana. The resulting conflict from this ethnic confrontation creates an upheavel that impacts the entire community.

Selena (1997) A biographical drama, this film presents the short life of Selena Quintanilla Perez, a charismatic Mexican-American Tejano singer. Selena was murdered in 1995 at the age of 23 by an ex-fan-club president. The movie contains many memorable scenes that portray life within Selena's loving, close-knit, and supportive Mexican-American family. The film also depicts the prejudice and condescending attitudes that confront Mexican-Americans. For example, when Selena enters a stylish dress shop and begins to try on clothes, the sales person automatically assumes that Selena (who is by now very wealthy) cannot afford to buy clothes in her shop because she is Mexican American.

Smoke Signals (1998) Based on *The Lone Ranger And Tonto Fist Fight In Heaven,* a 1995 collection of short stories by Sherman Alexie, *Smoke Signals* was written, directed, and produced by Native Americans. It tells about the journey of two young Native American men from the reservation to Phoenix, Arizona to claim one of the father's ashes. *Smoke Signals* won a major prize at the prestigious Sundance Film Festival.

Sunchaser (1996) A cultural clash arises when a privileged white male oncologist is forced to treat a dying half-Navaho called Blue, who is a convicted murderer. Blue forces the doctor to drive him to a mountaintop in Arizona where he can seek the help of a medicine man and cure his cancer by swimming in a magical, healing lake. As the physician and the young Navajo cross the desert together in search of spiritual healing, they eventually bond and come to see each other in a new light.

The Defiant Ones (1958) This Academy Award winning film tells the story of two convicts—one black and one white—who escape from a Southern prison. Shackled together, the convicts initially hate and distrust each other, but must learn to work together in order to survive. As the two men deal with escalating difficulties, they develop a respect for each other.

The Joy Luck Club (1993) Based on the successful 1989 novel by Amy Tan, this film blends eight stories and numerous flashbacks to portray the turbulent lives of four brave Chinese women who survived China's pre-World War II, male-dominated culture. The film depicts the women's immigration to the United States, and it explores their complex relationships with their four American-born daughters.

Witness (1985) A complex film with many layers, *Witness* is a detective story, a love story, and a transcultural portrait of the dramatic differences between Amish and mainstream American values. A young Amish boy on a journey with his mother witnesses a murder. Through a series of misadventures, the police detective assigned to the case is wounded, and the Amish community takes him in and hides him from the gunman. The young mother nurses the detective back to health, and during this process, the two fall in love. The young woman is warned by her alarmed father that she risks being shunned by the community if she continues her involvement with the detective. By the end of the film, the detective has solved the murder mystery, and he sadly leaves the Amish woman he loves, and the unyielding traditions of the Amish community, behind him.

APPENDIX

III

ANSWER KEY TO TESTING YOUR KNOWLEDGE QUESTIONS

Chapter 1: Introduction to Transcultural Communication

1. b. dyad
2. d. all of the above
3. b. decreased
4. a. increased
5. c. 30 million people

Chapter 2: Transcultural Communication Building Blocks: Culture, and Cultural Values

1. a. white, mainstream American culture
2. b. Japanese
3. d. all of the above
4. b. Amish
5. c. the Philippines
6. c. Iranian culture
7. d. Ultra-orthodox traditionalists

Chapter 3: Transcultural Communication Building Blocks: Beliefs, Behavior and Communication

1. c. utilizes such elements as yin and yang
2. b. extensive questioning, and the use of examination and laboratory techniques
3. b. emotional expressiveness
4. d. 40% of respondents
5. b. white North American
6. b. 18 inches to 4 feet

Chapter 4: Transcultural Communication Stumbling Blocks

1. d. all of the above
2. c. ethnocentrism

3. b. stereotyping
4. c. cultural blind spot syndrome
5. c. ritualistic

Chapter 5: Transcultural Communication Within The Health Care Subculture

1. a. hospital subculture conflict
2. b. professional subculture conflict
3. d. Western biomedical culture conflict
4. c. client subculture
5. d. all of the above
6. d. laughter, anger, and/or shock when encountering a therapy that is new or different

Chapter 6: Exploring Transcultural Communication as a Participant–Observer

1. c. selective inattention
2. d. complete participants
3. a. complete observer
4. c. participant-as-observer
5. a. broad-based, grand tour questions
6. c. is knowledgeable about the situation

Chapter 7: Using Basic Transcultural Communication Techniques

1. d. all of the above
2. b. Orientation Phase
3. c. informative rather than advising
4. b. lean slightly toward the client throughout the conversation
5. a. mirroring the client's communication style
6. c. position yourself parallel to and lower than the client

297

Chapter 8: Overcoming Transcultural Communication Barriers

1. b. dual ethnocentrism
2. b. a cultural stereotype
3. c. listen to the terms your client uses, and use those terms when communicating with the client instead of medical terms
4. d. all of the above

Chapter 9: Working With and Without An Interpreter

1. b. question the client via an interpreter
2. d. all of the above
3. c. Interpretation takes spoken words from one language and renders them in another language
4. c. maintain eye contact with the client, and address the client when asking questions
5. b. should not give a word-by-word interpretation, but should convey the intended idea of the client or professional

Chapter 10: Eliciting Assessment Data From The Client, Family, and Interpreters

1. d. expert healthcare professionals are able to intuit what questions to ask, and they know what feels right
2. b. believe that it is not necessary to conduct a cultural assessment on a client who is from the same cultural background
3. c. the client's explanation of illness.
4. b. an introduction and an indirect line of questioning followed by a handshake
5. d. all of the above
6. b. a linear pattern of care seeking
7. d. all of the above

Chapter 11: Using Transcultural Communication To Plan Care, Explain, and Instruct

1. b. listen, explain, and acknowledge differences
2. d. all of the above
3. d. fine tune your care plan so that it accommodates your client's cultural values and beliefs
4. b. right to refuse treatment without a reason
5. c. Mr. Gonzales will be able to list foods, seasonings, and beverages that are high in sodium and that are not allowed on his diet

Chapter 12: Using Transcultural Communication To Assist People Responding To Pain Grief, Dying, and Death

1. a. client's report of their perception of pain
2. b. pain threshold
3. c. death-denying
4. b. Mexican Americans
5. b. Japanese Americans
6. c. Mexican Americans
7. b. appropriate death

Chapter 13: Fostering Transcultural Communication With Other Health Care Professionals

1. c. unlicensed ancillary personnel
2. c. believe care providers should do everything to save a person's life
3. d. all of the above
4. d. Provide your supervisor with a written report of dates and incidents
5. c. arbitration

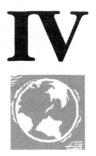

BIBLIOGRAPHY

Books

Agar, M. (1997). *The professional stranger: An informed introduction to ethnography.* 2nd ed. New York: Academic Press.

Aiken, T. D. with Catalano, J. T. (1994). *Legal, ethical, and political issues in nursing.* Philadelphia: Davis.

American heritage concise dictionary. 3rd ed. (1994). New York: Houghton Mifflin.

Andrews, M. M., & Boyle, J. S. (Eds.), (1998). *Transcultural concepts in nursing care.* 3rd ed. Philadelphia: Lippincott.

Axtell, R. E. (Ed.), (1993). *Do's and taboos around the world.* 3rd ed. New York: Wiley.

Bailey, E. J. (1991). *Urban African American health care.* Indianapolis: University Press of America.

Barnhart, D. K. & Metcalf, A. (1997). *America in so many words: Words that have shaped America.* Boston: Houghton Mifflin.

Benner, P. (1984). *From novice to expert.* Menlo Park, CA: Addison-Wesley.

Bolander, V. B. (1994). *Sorenson & Luckmann's basic nursing: A psychophysiologic approach.* 3rd ed. Philadelphia: Saunders.

Bongard, E. S. & Darryl, S. Y. (Ed.) (1993). *Current critical care diagnosis and treatment.* East Norwalk, CT: Appleton & Lange.

Burgess, A. W. (1997). *Psychiatric nursing: Promoting mental health.* Stamford, CT: Appleton & Lange.

Ellis, J. R. & Hartley, C. L. (1995). *Managing and coordinating nursing care.* 2nd ed. Philadelphia: Lippincott.

Fetterman, D. M. (1998). *Ethnography: Step by step.* Thousand Oaks, CA: Sage.

Giger, J. N. & Davidhizar, R. E. (1999). *Transcultural nursing: Assessment and intervention.* 3rd ed. St. Louis: Mosby.

Gropper, R. (1996). *Culture and the clinical encounter: An intercultural sensitizer for the health professions.* Yarmouth, ME: Intercultural Press.

Hunter, D. E. & Foley, M. B. (1976). *Doing anthropology: A student-centered approach to cultural anthropology.* New York: Harper & Row.

Jamieson, D. & O'Mara, J. (1991). *Managing workforce 2000: Gaining the diversity advantage.* San Francisco: Josey Bass.

Laungani, P. (1992). *It shouldn't happen to a patient.* London: Whiting & Birch.

Lee, E. (Ed.), (1997). *Working with Asian Americans: A guide for clinicians.* San Francisco: Richman Area Multi-Services, Inc.

Leininger, M. (1978). *Transcultural nursing: Theories, concepts, and practices.* New York: Wiley.

Lipson, J., Dibble, S. & Minarik, P. (1996). *Culture & nursing care: A pocket guide.* San Francisco: UCSF Nursing Press.

Luckmann, J. (Ed.). (1997). *Saunder's manual of nursing care.* Philadelphia: Saunders.

Morse, J. M. & Field, P. A. (1995). *Qualitative research methods for health professionals.* Thousand Oaks, CA: Sage.

Paniagua, F. A. (1999). *Assessing and treating culturally diverse clients.* 2nd ed. Thousand Oaks, CA: Sage.

Pedersen, P. (1988). *A handbook for developing multicultural awareness.* Alexandria, VA: American Association for Counseling and Development.

Perkins, J., Simon, H., Cheng, F., Olson, K., & Vera, Y. (1998). *Ensuring linguistic access in health care settings: Legal rights and responsibilities.* Menlo Park, California: National Health Law Program for the Henry J. Kaiser Family Foundation.

Purnell, L. D. & Paulanka, B. J. (1998). *Transcultural health care: A culturally competent approach.* Philadelphia: Davis.

Rando, T. A. (1984). *Grief, Dying, and Death.* Champaign, IL.: Research Press. pp. 1–41.

Scrimshaw, S. C. M. & Hurtado, E. (1987). *Rapid assessment procedures for nutrition and primary health care.* Los Angeles: UCLA Latin American Center Publications.

Singelis, T. M. (Ed). (1998). *Teaching about culture, ethnicity, and diversity: Exercises and planned activities.* Thousands Oaks, CA: Sage.

Smitherman, G. (1994). *Black talk: Words and phrases from the hood to the amen corner.* Boston: Houghton Mifflin.

Spradley, J. P. (1979). *The ethnographic interview.* New York: Holt, Rinehart & Winston.

Spradley, J. P. (1980). *Participant observation.* New York: Holt, Rinehart & Winston.

Sue, D. W. & Sue, D. (1999). *Counseling the culturally different: Theory and practice.* 3rd ed. New York: Wiley.

Terrance, O. (1994). *Comprehensive accreditation manual for hospitals 1995.* Joint Commission of Accreditation of Healthcare Organizations.

Thelan, L. A., Urden, L. D., Lough, M. E., & Stacey, K. M. (1997). *Critical care nursing: Diagnosis and management.* 2nd ed. St. Louis: Mosby.

Townsend, M. C. (1996). *Psychiatric mental health nursing: Concepts of care.* 2nd ed. Philadelphia: Davis.

Williams, R. L. (1975). *Ebonics: The true language of black folks.* St. Louis: Institute of Black Studies. (This book was based on papers submitted by Robert L. Williams in 1973).

Worden, J. W. (1982). *Grief counseling and grief therapy.* New York: Springer.

Zehavi, A. M. (Ed.), (1973). *Handbook of the world's religions.* New York: Franklin Watts.

Articles, Pamphlets, and Book Chapters

Alternative medicine: Separating fact from fiction. (1994). *The University of Texas Lifetime Health Letter.* 6(5):1, 6.

American Demographics Inc., (1991). American diversity: What the 1990 census reveals about population growth, blacks, Hispanics, Asians, ethnic diversity, and children—and what it means to you. *American Demographics Desk Reference Series.* No 1.

Anderson, K. (1983). Los Angeles: America's uneasy new melting pot. *Time.* pp. 18–25.

Andrea, J. & Renner, P. (1996). Interpreting the needs of the ED patient: One California hospital's 3 week study. *Emergency Nursing.* 21(6):510–512.

Andrews, M. M. & Boyle, J. S. (1997). Competence in transcultural nursing. *American Journal of Nursing.* 97(8): 16AAA–16DDD.

Associated Press. (1997, August 1). Medical interpreters decry budget cuts. *Seattle Post-Intelligencier.* B-3.

Avery, C. (1991). Native American medicine: Traditional healing. *Journal of the American Medical Association.* 265(17):2271–2273.

Banks, L. J. (1992). Counseling. In Bulechek, G. M. & McCloskey, J. C. *Nursing Intervention.* 2nd Ed. 279–291.

Barbee, E. L. (1993). Racism in U.S. nursing. *Medical Anthropology Quarterly.* 7(4):346–362.

Battaglia, B. (1998). Cultural views on death and dying...part 3. *Cross Cultural Connection.* 3(3):1–4.

Brewer, J. A. & Bonalumi, N. M. (1996). Cultural diversity in the emergency department: Health care beliefs and practices among the Pennsylvania Amish. *Journal of Emergency Nursing.* 21(6):494–497.

Brink, P. J. (1990). Cultural diversity in the nursing profession. In McCluskey, J. C. & Grace, H. K. (Eds.). *Current Issues in Nursing.* 3rd ed. Boston: Blackwell Scientific. pp. 935–939.

Buchwald, D., et al. (1994). Caring for patients in a multicultural society. *Patient Care.* 28(11):105–123.

Burner, O. Y., et al. (1990). Managing a multicultural nurse staff in a multicultural environment. *Journal of Nursing Administration.* 20(6):30–34.

Bushy, A. (1992). Cultural considerations for primary health care: Where do self-care and folk medicine fit? *Holistic Nurse Practitioner.* 6(3):10–18.

Campinha-Bacote, J. (1995). The quest for cultural competence in nursing care. *Nursing Forum.* 30(4):19–25.

Campinha-Bacote, J. (1998). African-Americans. In Purnell, L. D. & Paulanka, B. J. *Transcultural Health Care: A Culturally Competent Approach.* Philadelphia: Davis.

Chalanda, M. (1995). Brokerage in multicultural nursing. *International Nursing Review.* 42(1):19–22, 26.

Charnes, L. S. (1992). Meeting patient's spiritual needs: The Jewish perspective. *Holistic Nurse Practitioner.* 6(3):64–72.

Charonko, D. V. (1992). Cultural influences in noncompliant behavior and decision making. *Holistic Nurse Practitioner.* 6(3):73–78.

Cherry, B. & Giger, J. N. (1999). African Americans In: Giger, J. N. & Davidhizar, R. E. (Eds.). *Transcultural Nursing: Assessment and Intervention.* 3rd ed. St. Louis: Mosby.

Chester, B. & Holtan, N. (1992). Working with refugee survivors of torture (Cross-cultural medicine—A decade later). *Western Journal of Medicine.* 157:301–304.

Cochran, M. M. (1998). Tears have no color: The medical world is not always prepared for the collision of cultures. *American Journal of Nursing.* 98(6):53.

Corr, C. A., Nabe, C. M., & Corr, D. M. (1994). *Death and Dying, Life and Living.* Pacific Grove, CA: Brooks/Cole. pp. 73–121.

Cowles, K.V. (1996). Cultural perspectives of grief: An expanded concept analysis. *Journal of Advanced Nursing.* 23, 287–294.

Cravener, P. (1992). Establishing therapeutic alliance across cultural barriers. *Journal of Psychosocial Nursing.* 30(12):10–14.

Daley, B. (1997). Therapeutic touch, nursing practice and contemporary cutaneous wound healing research. *Journal of Advanced Nursing.* 25(6): 1123–1132.

Davidhizar, R. & Giger, J. N. (1994). When your patient is silent. *Journal of Advanced Nursing.* 20(4):703–706.

Davidhizar, R., et al. (1997). Model for cultural diversity in the radiology department. *Radiologic Technology.* 68(3):233–238.

Delk-Calkins, K. (1984). What to do until the translator arrives. *Journal of Practical Nursing.* 34(2):12–13, 61.

DeSantis, L. (1994). Making anthropology clinically relevant to nursing care. *Journal of Advanced Nursing.* 20(4):707–715.

Dinh, H. (1997). Translation initiative. *Contemporary Nurse.* 6(2):75–76.

Dossey, B. M. & Dossey, L. (1998). Attending to holistic care. *American Journal of Nursing.* 98(8):35–38.

Doswell, W. M. (1998). Multicultural issues and ethical concerns in the delivery of nursing care interventions. *Nursing Clinics of North America.* 33(2): 353–361.

Easter, A. (1997). The state of research on the effects of therapeutic touch. *Journal of Holistic Nursing.* 15(2):158–175.

Edmission, K. W. (1997). Psychosocial dimensions of medical-surgical nursing. In Black, J. M. & Matassarin-Jacobs, E. (Eds.). *Medical Surgical Nursing: Clinical Management for Continuity of Care.* Philadelphia: Saunders.

Eng, J. L. Health workers trying to bridge cultural gaps: Study explores ethnic differences in approaching death and dying. (1998, October 18). *The Seattle Times.* B8.

Evans, C. A. & Cunningham, B. A. (1996). Caring for the ethnic elder. *Geriatric Nursing.* 17(3):105–110.

Fairlie, A. (1992). Nurse–patient communication barriers. *Senior Nurse.* 12(3):40–43.

Fein, E. B. (1997, November 23). Language barriers are hindering health care. *The New York Times.* p. 20.

Felstiner, W. L. F., et al. (1981). The emergence and transformation of disputes: Naming, blaming, claiming. *Law Sociology Review.* 15(34):631–654.

Fielo, S. B. & Degazon, C. E. (1997). When cultures collide: Decision making in a multicultural environment. *Nursing and Health Care Perspectives.* 18(5):238–243.

Fong, C. M. (1985). Ethnicity and nursing practice. *Topics in Clinical Nursing.* 7(3):1–10.

Foong, A. (1992). Challenging the tower of Babel: The increasing diversity in cultures. *Nursing.* 5(5):12–25.

Fryback, P. B. & Reinert, B. R. (1997). Alternative therapies and control for health in cancer and AIDS. *Clinical Nurse Specialist.* 11(2):64–69.

Gannett Service. (1994, January 19). Many don't use English at home. *San Antonio Express News,* 18A.

Gary, F. A., Sigsby, L. M. & Campbell, D. (1998). Preparing for the 21st century: Diversity in nursing education, research, and practice. *Journal of Professional Nursing.* 14(5):272–279.

Geissler, F. M. (1992). Nursing diagnoses: A study of cultural relevance. *Journal of Professional Nursing.* 8(5):301–307.

Germain, C. P. (1992). Cultural care: A bridge between sickness, illness, and disease. *Holistic Nurse Practitioner.* 6(3):1–9.

Germain, C. P. (1993). Ethnography: The method. In Munhall, P. L. & Boyd, C. O. (Eds). *Nursing Research: A Qualitative Perspective.* New York: National League for Nursing Press. pp. 237–268.

Gibbs, R. D. et al. (1987). Patient understanding of commonly used medical vocabulary. *Journal of Family Practice.* 25(2):176–178.

Giger, J. N. & Davidhizar, R. J. (1990). Transcultural nursing assessment: A method for advancing nursing practice. *International Nursing Review.* 37(1):199–202.

Giger, J. N. & Davidhizar, R. J. (1996). When the operating room has a multicultural team. *Today's Surgical Nurse.* 18(5):26–32.

Gordon, C. (1997). The effect of cancer pain on quality of life in different ethnic groups: A literature review. *Nurse Practitioner Forum.* 3(1):5–13.

Grossman, D. (1996). Cultural dimensions in home health nursing. *American Journal of Nursing.* 96(7):33–36.

Haffner, L. (1992). Translation is not enough: Interpreting in a medical setting. (*Cross-Cultural Medicine—A Decade Later*) Special Issue. *Western Journal of Medicine.* 157 (special issue): pp. 328–332.

Hagland, M. M. (1993). Crossing cultures: hospitals begin breaking down the barriers to care. *Hospitals.* 67:29.

Harris, L. H. & Tuck, I. (1992). The role of the organization and nurse manager in integrating transcultural concepts into nursing practice. *Holistic Nurse Practitioner.* 6(3):43–48.

Hatton, D. C. (1992). Information transmission in bilingual, bicultural contexts. *Journal of Community Health Nursing.* 9(1):53–59.

Hatton, D. C. (1993). Information transmission in bilingual, bicultural contexts: A field study of community health nurses and interpreters. *Journal of Community Health Nursing.* 10(3):137–147.

Herberg, P. (1998). Theoretical foundations of transcultural nursing. In Andrews, M. M. & Boyle, J. S. (Eds.). *Transcultural Concepts in Nursing Care.* 3rd ed. Philadelphia: Lippincott.

Hiok-Boon Lin, E. (1983). Intraethnic characteristics and the patient-physician interaction: "Cultural blind spot syndrome." *The Journal of Family Practice.* 16(1):91–98.

Holmes, S. A. (1998). Blacks consider new face of race issues. *Seattle Times.* 47.

Hughes, O. M. (1997). Caring for people in pain. In Luckmann, J. (Ed.). *Saunder's Manual of Nursing Care.* Philadelphia: Saunders.

Jackson, L. E. (1993). Understanding, eliciting, and negotiating client's multicultural health beliefs. *Nurse Practitioner.* 18(4):30–43.

Jackson, M. The black experience with death: A brief analysis through black writings. In Kalish, R. A. (Ed.). (1980). *Death and Dying: Views From Many Cultures.* New York: Baywood. pp. 92–97.

Jein, R. F. & Harris, B. L. (1989). Cross-cultural conflict: The American nurse manager and a culturally mixed staff. *Journal of the New York State Nurses Association.* 20(2):16–19.

Jezewski, M. A. (1990). Culture brokering in migrant farmworkers care. *Western Journal of Nursing Research.* 12(4):497–513.

Jones, M. E., Bond, M. L. & Mancini, M. E. (1998). Developing a culturally competent work force: An opportunity for collaboration. *Journal of Professional Nursing.* 15(5):187–280.

Kaufert, J. M. (1997). Communication through interpreters in healthcare: Ethical dilemmas arising from differences in class, culture, language, and power. *Journal of Clinical Ethics.* 8(1):71–87.

Keegan, L. (1998). Getting comfortable with alternative and complementary therapies. *Nursing 98.* 28(4):50–53.

King, W. (1994, September 20). Book on alternative medicine stirs ill will. *The Seattle Times,* Section B, pp. 1, 2.

Kirkham, S. R. (1998). Nurses' descriptions of caring for culturally diverse clients. *Clinical Nursing Research.* 7(2):125–146.

Klessig, J. (1992). Cross-cultural medicine: A decade later. *Western Journal of Medicine.* 157(3):316–322.

Klessig, J. (1992). The effect of values and culture in life-support decisions. *Western Journal of Medicine.* 177(3):316–322.

Kotora, J. (1997). Therapeutic touch can augment traditional therapies. In Knobf, M. T. & Donovan, C. T. (Eds.). Practice corner. Practice tips from the Yale Cancer Center, New Haven, CT. *Oncology Nursing Forum.* 24(8): 1329–1330.

Kramer, M. (1968). Role models, role conceptions, and role deprivation. *Nursing Research.* 17(2):115–120.

Kramer, M. (1970). Role conceptions of baccalaureate nurses and success in hospital nursing. *Nursing Research.* 19(5):428–439.

Kumasaka, L. (1996). "My pain is God's will." *American Journal of Nursing.* 96(6):45–47.

Lajkowicz, C. (1993). Teaching cultural diversity for the workplace. *Journal of Nursing Education.* 32(5):235–236.

Landmark Healthcare (1998). *The Landmark report on public perceptions of alternative care.* Sacramento, CA: Landmark Healthcare.

Lapierre, E. D. & Padgett, J. (1991). How can we become more aware of culturally specific body language and use this awareness therapeutically? *Journal of Psychosocial Nursing.* 29(11):38–41.

Lau, J. (1998). A survey of multicultural awareness among hospital and clinical staff. [letter]. *Journal of Nursing Care Quality.* 12(4):67–69.

Lawson, L. V. (1990). Culturally sensitive support for grieving parents. *American Journal of Maternal/Child Nursing.* 15(2):76–79.

Leap, N. (1992). The power of words. *Nursing Times.* 88(21):60–61.

Lefever, D. & Davidhizar, R. E. (1999). American Eskimos. In Giger, J. N. & Davidhizer, R. E. (Eds.). *Transcultural Nursing: Assessment and Intervention.* 3rd ed. St. Louis: Mosby.

Leininger, M. (1996). Founder's focus. Transcultural nurses and consumers tell their stories. *Journal of Transcultural Nursing.* 7(2):32–36.

Leininger, M. (1996). Transcultural nursing administration: An imperative worldwide. *Journal of Transcultural Nursing.* 8(1):28–33.

Leininger, M. (1997). Understanding cultural pain for improved health care. *Journal of Transcultural Nursing.* 9(1):32–35.

Lester, N. (1998). Cultural competence: A nursing dialogue. *American Journal of Nursing.* 98(8):26–34.

Lester, N. (1998). Cultural competence: A nursing dialogue. (Part II). *American Journal of Nursing.* 98(9):36–44.

Lim, D. (1997). Culture and advance directives. *American Nephrology Nurses' Association Journal.* 24(1):69, 97.

Lipson, J. G. (1992). The health and adjustment of Iranian immigrants. *Western Journal of Nursing Research.* 14(1):10–29.

Lipson, J. G. & Hafizi, H. (1998). Iranians. In Purnell, L. D. & Paulanka, B. J. (Eds.). *Transcultural Health Care: A Culturally Competent Approach.* Philadelphia: Davis.

Lowenstein, A. J. & Glanville, C. (1991). Transcultural concepts applied to nursing administration. *Journal of Nursing Administration.* 21(3):13–14.

Lowenstein, A. J. & Glanville, C. (1995). Cultural diversity and conflict in the health care workplace. *Nursing Economics.* 13(4):203–209.

Ludwig-Beymer, P. (1998). Transcultural aspects of pain. In Andrews, M. M. & Boyle, J. S. *Transcultural Concepts in Nursing Care.* Philadelphia: Lippincott.

Magnus, M. H. (1996). What's your IQ on cross-cultural nutrition counseling? *The Diabetes Educator.* 22(1):57–60.

Mailhot, C. B. (1997). Culture and consent. *Nursing Management.* 28(3):48.

Malone, B. L. (1993). Caring for culturally diverse racial groups: An administrative matter. *Nursing Administration Quarterly.* 17(2):21–29.

Martin, C. (1999). Irish Americans. In Giger, J. N. & Davidhizar, R. E. (Eds.). *Transcultural Nursing: Assessment and Intervention.* 3rd ed. St. Louis: Mosby.

Matsumoto, D. (1989). Face, culture, and judgments of anger and fear: Do the eyes have it? *Journal of Nonverbal Behavior.* 13:171–188.

Mattson, S. & Johnson, L. (1992). Integration of cultural content into a psychiatric nursing course to change students' attitudes and decrease anxiety. *Nurse Educator.* 17(4):5.

Mauksch, L. B. & Roesler, T. (1990). Expanding the context of the patient's explanatory model using circular questioning. *Family Systems Medicine.* 8(1):3–13.

McArthur, J. H. & Moore, F. D. (1997). The two cultures and the health care revolution. *Journal of the American Medical Association.* 277(12):985–989.

Meadows, J. L. (1991). Multicultural communication. Sections of this paper were presented at a Maternal and Child Health Conference on *The*

Meaning of Culture in Health Care at the University of Illinois at Chicago College of Associated Health Professions.

Meadows, J. L. (1991). Multicultural communication. *The Hawthorne Press.* pp. 31–42.

Meleis, A. I. (1997). Immigrant transitions and health care: An action plan [News]. *Nursing Outlook.* 45(1):42.

Melzack, R. & Wall, P. D. (1965). Pain mechanism: A new theory. *Science.* 150(36):971–972.

Miller, S. W. & Goodin, J. N. (1995). East Indian Hindu Americans. In Giger, J. N. & Davidhizar, R. E. (Eds.). *Transcultural nursing: Assessment and Intervention.* 2nd ed. St. Louis: Mosby.

Miranda, B. F., McBride, M. R. & Spangler, Z. (1998). Filipino Americans. In Purnell, L. D. & Paulanka, B. J. (Eds.). *Transcultural Health Care: A Culturally Competent Approach.* Philadelphia: Davis.

Morgan, B. S. (1984). A semantic differential measure of attitudes toward black American patients. *Research in Nursing and Health.* 7:155–172.

Morganthau, T. (1995). What color is black? *Newsweek.* 125(7):62–69.

Murphy, F. G., Anderson, R. M. & Lyons, A. E. (1993). Diabetes educators as cultural translators. *The Diabetes Educator.* 19(2):13–18.

Narayan, M. C. (1997). Cultural assessment in home health care. *Home Health Care Nurse.* 15(10):663–670.

Newman, J. (1998). Managing cultural diversity: The art of communication. *Radiographic Technology.* 69(3):231–246, 249.

Nichter, M. & Nichter, M. (1996). Education by appropriate analogy. In Nichter, M. and Nichter, M. (Eds.). *Anthropology and International Health: Asian Case Studies.* 2nd ed. The Netherlands: Gordon and Breach, pp. 400–425.

Pacquiao, D. F. (1995). Multicultural issues in nursing practice and education. *Newsletter of the National Council of State Boards of Nursing.* 16(2):1, 4, 5, 11.

Perry, H. L. (1993). Mourning and funeral customs of African Americans. In Irish, B. O., Jenkins, J. E., & Lundquist, B. L., (Eds.). *Ethnic Variations in Dying, Death, and Grief: Diversity in Universality.* Washington, DC: Taylor & Francis. pp. 51–65.

Pickett, M. (1993). Cultural awareness in the context of terminal illness. *Cancer Nursing.* 16(2):102–106.

Pliskin, K. L. (1992). Dysphoria and somatization in Iranian culture (Cross-cultural medicine—A decade later). Special Issue. *The Western Journal of Medicine.* 157:295–300.

Porter, C. P. & Villarruel, A. M. (1993). Nursing research with African American and Hispanic people: Guidelines for action. *Nursing Outlook.* 41(2):59–67.

Price, J. L. & Cordell, B. (1994). Cultural diversity and patient teaching. *The Journal of Continuing Education in Nursing.* 25(4):163–166.

Purnell, L. D. & Paulanka, B. J. (1998). Purnell's model for cultural competence. In Purnell, L. D. & Paulanka, B. J. (Eds.). *Transcultural Health Care: A Culturally Competent Approach.* Philadelphia: Davis.

Puterbaugh, S. (1991). Communicating when the patient cannot speak English. *Today's OR Nurse.* 13(1)31.

Putsch, R. W. (1985). Cross-cultural communication: The special case of interpreters in health care. *Journal of the American Medical Association.* 254 (23):3344–3348.

Rader, G. S. (1988, July). Management decisions: Do we really need interpreters? *Nursing Management.* 19(7):46–48.

Roat, C. E. (1997). A medical interpreter's code of ethics. In Roat, C. E. (ed.). *Bridging the Gap: A Basic Training for Medical Interpreters: Trainer's Curriculum.* Seattle, WA: Cross-Cultural Health Care Program. pp. 34–35.

Rosella, J. D. et al. (1994). The need for multicultural diversity among health professionals. *Nursing and Health Care.* 15(5):242–246.

Rosenbaun, J. N. (1991). A cultural assessment guide: Learning cultural sensitivity. *The Canadian Nurse.* 87(4):32–33.

Ross, H. M. (1981). Societal/cultural views regarding death and dying. *Topics in Clinical Nursing.* pp. 1–13.

Rothenburger, R. L. (1990). Transcultural nursing: Overcoming obstacles to effective communication. *AORN Journal.* 51(5):1349–1363.

Sabatino, F. (1993). Culture shock: Are U. S. hospitals ready? *Hospitals.* 67(1): 22–25, 28–31.

Salerno, E. (1995). Race, culture, and medications. *Journal of Emergency Nursing.* 21(6):560–562.

Schwartz, E. A. (1999). Jewish Americans. In Giger, J. N. & Davidhizar, R. E. (Eds.). *Transcultural Nursing: Assessment and Intervention.* 3rd ed. St. Louis: Mosby.

Scrimshaw, S. C. M. & Hurtado, E. (1984). Field guide for the study of health seeking behavior at the household level. *Food and Nutrition Bulletin.* 6(2):27–45.

Selekman, J. (1998). Jewish Americans. In Purnell, L. D. & Paulanka, B. J. (Eds.). *Transcultural Health Care: A Culturally Competent Approach.* Philadelphia: Davis.

Setness, P. A. (1998). Culturally competent healthcare. *Postgraduate Medicine.* 103(2):13–16.

Sherer, J. L. (1993). Crossing cultures: Hospitals begin breaking down the barriers to care. *Hospitals.* 67(1):22–25, 28–31.

Snyder, J. R. (1997). Complementary therapies in hospice care. Therapeutic touch and the terminally ill: Healing power through the hands. *American Journal of Hospice and Palliative Care.* 14(2):83–87.

Souminen, T., et al. (1997). Nursing culture—some viewpoints. *Journal of Advanced Nursing.* 25(1):186–190.

Spangler, A. (1992). Transcultural care values and practices of Philippine-American nurses. *Journal of Transcultural Nursing.* 4(2):13–28.

Stewart, M. (1998). Nurses need to strengthen cultural competence for next century to ensure quality patient care. *American Nurse.* 30(1):26–27.

Stokes, L. G. (1977). Delivering health services in a Black community. In: Reinhardt, A. M. & Quinn, M. B. (Eds.). *Current Practice In Family-Centered Community Nursing.* St. Louis: Mosby.

Sutherland, D. & Morris, B. J. (1996). Caring for the Islamic patient. *Journal of Emergency Nursing.* 21(6):508–509.

Thiederman, S. B. (1986). Ethnocentrism: A barrier to effective health care. *Nurse Practitioner.* 11(8):52–59.

Tilki, M., et al. (1994). Learning from colleagues of different cultures. *British Journal of Nursing.* 3(21):1118–1124.

Tips for overcoming cultural barriers. (1998). *Same-Day Surgery.* 22(4):Supplement 4.

Toumishey, L. H. (1989). Strangers among strangers: Clients and health practitioners in health care settings. *Nurse Education Today.* 9(6):363–367.

To work with culturally diverse patients, tailor lessons to individual. *Patient Education Management.* (1998) 5(3):29–32, 44.

Tripp-Reimer, T. & Afifi, L. A. (1989). Cross-cultural perspectives on patient teaching. *Nursing Clinics of North America.* 24(3):613–619.

Trossman, S. (1998). Diversity: A continuing challenge. *American Nurse.* 30(1): 1,24–25.

Ulrich, L. P. (1994). The Patient Self-Determination Act and cultural diversity. *Cambridge Quarterly of Healthcare Ethics.* 3(3):410–413.

Vance, A. R. (1999). Filipino Americans. In Giger, J. N. & Davidhizar, R. E. (Eds.). *Transcultural Nursing: Assessment and Intervention.* 3rd ed. St. Louis: Mosby.

Villaire, M. (1994). Interview with Toni Tripp-Reimer: Crossing over the boundaries. *Critical Care Nurse.* pp. 134–141.

Villarruel, A. M. & de Montellano, B. O. (1992). Culture and pain: A meso-American perspective. *Advanced Nursing Science.* 15(1):21–32.

Walker, A. C., Tan, L. & George, S. (1995). Impact of culture on pain management: An Australian nursing perspective. *Holistic Nursing Practice.* 9(2):48–57.

Walton, J. C. & Waszkiewiez, M. (1997). Managing unlicensed assistive personnel: Tips for improving quality outcomes. *Medsurg Nursing.* 6(1): 124–128.

Weber, S. E. (1996). Cultural aspects of pain in childbearing women. *JOGNN.* 25(1):67–72.

Wenger, A. F. Z. (1991). Culture-specific care and the Old Order Amish. *NSNA Imprint.* pp. 80–93.

Wenger, A. F. Z. (1993). Cultural meaning of symptoms. *Holistic Nurse Practitioner.* 7(2):22–35.

Wenger, A. F. Z. & Wenger, M. R. (1998). The Amish. In Purnell, L. D. & Paulanka, B. J. (Eds.). *Transcultural Health Care: A Culturally Competent Approach.* Philadelphia: Davis.

Williams, J. & Rodgers, S. (1993). The multicultural workplace: Preparing preceptors. *The Journal of Continuing Education in Nursing.* 24(3):101–104

Wilson, S. A. (1998). Irish-Americans. In Purnell, L. D. & Paulanka, B. J. (Eds.). *Transcultural Health Care: A Culturally Competent Approach.* Philadelphia: Davis.

Wright, F., et al. (1997). Diverse decisions: How culture affects ethical decision making. *Nursing Clinics of North America.* 9(1):63–74.

Younoszai, B. (1993). Mexican American perspectives related to death. In Irish, D. P., Lundquist, K. F., & Nelson, V. J. (Eds.). *Ethnic Variations in Dying, Death, and Grief: Diversity in Universality.* Washington, DC.: Taylor & Francis. pp. 67–99.

Zatzick, D. F. & Dimsdale, J. (1990). Cultural variations in response to painful stimuli. *Psychosomatic Medicine.* pp. 52, 544–557.

Zich, A. (1991). Japan's sun rises over the Pacific. *National Geographic.* pp. 35–66.

Media

Compton's Interactive Encyclopedia. Copyright © 1994, 1995, 1996. Compton's NewMedia, Inc.

Intuit. *Microsoft® Encarta® Encyclopedia* © 1993–1996. Microsoft Corporation. All rights reserved.

Microsoft (1996). *Microsoft Encarta 97 Encyclopedia.* Microsoft Corporation.

Native Americans. *Microsoft® Encarta® Encyclopedia* © 1993–1996. Microsoft Corporation. All rights reserved.

Government Publications

1990 U.S. Census and the Sourcebook of Zipcode Demographics.

1990 Census of population. Social and economic characteristics, United States Bureau of the Census, Washington, DC: U. S. Printing Office, 15, 1990.

California Health and Safety Code, Section 1259 (Daring's Supplement, 1995).

Title 45 Code of Federal Regulations, Part 80—Nondiscrimination under programs receiving federal assistance through the Department of Health and Human Services effectuation of Title VI of the Civil Rights Act of 1964. Department of Health and Human Services, 45 CFRA (10-1-94 Edition), pp. 292–293.

U. S. Department of Commerce, Economic, and Statistics Administration Bureau of the Census. *Statistical Abstract of the U. S.: The National Data book.* 1996.

U. S. Department of Health and Human Services Public Health Services. *Acute Pain Management: Clinical Practice Guidelines.* AHCPR Pub. No. 92-0032 Rockville, MD: Agency for Health Care Policy and Research. February, 1992.

Personal Communications

Letter from Cynthia Roat, Interpreter Training Coordinator, Cross-Cultural Health Care Program at PacMed Clinics in Seattle, Washington, July 25, 1995.

Telephone Conference with Cynthia Roat, Interpreter Training Coordinator, Cross-Cultural Health Care Program at PacMed Clinics in Seattle, Washington, June 12, 1998.

Unpublished Papers

Dreyfus, S. & Dreyfus, H. (1980). A five-stage model of the mental activities involved in directed skill acquisition. Unpublished Report. University of California at Berkeley.

INDEX

313